Basic Telecommunications for Emergency Medical Services

Basic Telecommunications for Emergency Medical Services

James E. McCorkle, Jr. P.E.
Eugene L. Nagel, M.D.
Brig. Gen. Donald G. Penterman (Ret.)
Robert A. Mason

Ballinger Publishing Company • Cambridge, Massachusetts
A Subsidiary of J.B. Lippincott Company

International Standard Book Number: 0–88410–703–5

Library of Congress Catalog Card Number: 77–27303

Printed in the United States of America

Library of Congress Cataloging in Publication Data

Main entry under title:

Basic telecommunications for emergency medical services.

"Based in part upon a report prepared . . . by the Communications Subcommittee of the Committee on Emergency Medical Services of the National Academy of Sciences."
1. Emergency medical services—Communication systems. I. McCorkle, James E. II. National Academy of Sciences. Committee on Emergency Medical Services. Communications Subcommittee. [DNLM: 1. Emergency health services. 2. Telecommunications. WX215 B311]
RA645.5.B37   362.1   77–27303
ISBN 0–88410–703–5

It is the wish of the working group to dedicate this volume to BRIG. GEN. SAM SEELEY (RET.), former staff associate, National Academy of Sciences, whose timely and effective efforts did much to focus national attention on the need for emergency medical services systems.

Contents

List of Figures

List of Tables

Foreword

When the Robert Wood Johnson Foundation became a national philanthropy in 1972, it made a commitment to assist Americans in gaining better access to general medical care. It was soon recognized that one particular problem citizens faced was the lack of prompt access to appropriate emergency medical services.

Thus, in April 1973, The Johnson Foundation announced the availability of $15 million on a competitive basis to assist communities in developing regional emergency medical communications systems. The program, which was jointly administered with the National Academy of Sciences, resulted in the awarding of forty-four grants to regions in thirty-two states and Puerto Rico.

In developing truly regional emergency medical communications systems, many of the barriers that confront communities have been organizational and political. Other significant barriers, however, are technical and include important issues relating to radio frequencies and the Federal Communications Commission. These communications issues were made even more complex by the important new FCC ruling in 1974 (Docket No. 19880) relating to emergency medical services. To provide communities with a better understanding of these new regulations, the Foundation, working with the American Medical Association, sponsored a series of regional workshops in 1974 and 1975 which addressed communications questions.

It was also apparent that no single report or document contained current and easily understandable information about emergency medical communications. Thus, the Foundation provided support to four nationally recognized experts in emergency medical services to enable them to prepare this book. Dr. David McConnaughey at the National Academy of Sciences provided valuable editorial assistance. The manuscript was also reviewed by several members of the National Academy of Sciences' Advisory Committee on emergency medical services and staff members of the Division of emergency medical services of the Department of Health, Education and Welfare.

This book should be of great value to communities throughout the country as they continue to develop and refine regional systems of emergency medical care.

Blair L. Sadler
Vice President
Director, Hospital & Clinics
Scripps Clinic and Research Foundation

(Formerly Assistant Vice President
The Robert Wood Johnson Foundation)

Foreword

The effective interconnection of the many elements comprising an emergency medical services system is a complex problem. The particular solution of such a problem must be placed on technology, properly applied, and suited to the region in question. In most cases the individual with background and understanding in EMS will not be the same person able to solve the problem in applied technology. Thus a communication problem arises between these individuals that is not addressed specifically within this volume. Instead the book itself is designed to facilitate communications between nontechnical and technical personnel working in EMS.

The Committee on Emergency Medical Services asked that this book be prepared to address the fundamental communications problem identified above. I believe that viewed from this perspective, BASIC TELECOMMUNICATIONS FOR EMERGENCY MEDICAL SERVICES offers an important contribution to the field of EMS.

Donald S. Gann, M.D.
Chairman, National Academy of Sciences
National Research Council
Committee on EMS

Preface

This work is based in part upon a report prepared during 1970–1972 by the Communications Subcommittee of the Committee on Emergency Medical Services of the National Academy of Sciences, under the sponsorship of the Department of Health, Education and Welfare and the Department of Transportation. At that time, developments in emergency medical communications equipment and in Federal Communications Commission regulations governing radio frequencies available for EMS systems were moving so rapidly that publication was deferred while the report was repeatedly revised.

Preparation of the study was made possible by the Robert Wood Johnson Foundation, and accomplished with the encouragement of the Division of Emergency Medical Services of HEW and the approval of the National Academy of Sciences. The work was performed chiefly by James E. McCorkle, Jr., P.E., in collaboration with Eugene L. Nagel, M.D., Brig. Gen. Donald Penterman, and Robert A. Mason, all members of the NAS Committee on Emergency Medical Services. Appreciation is expressed for the valuable assistance given by the late Art Griffiths, HEW/EMS, and to David McConnaughey, NAS/ ALS, for suggestions and assistance.

Introduction

The purpose of this book is to provide noncommunications personnel involved in developing a regional Emergency Medical Services (EMS) system with a general understanding of the application, design, and implementation of a supporting EMS communication system. The functions that communications must serve at each operational step of the EMS system will be defined, and the information needed by the communication specialist to draw up a detailed communication plan, with equipment specifications, will be provided.

It should be recognized at the outset that communication system is a resource only. It can, however, be a necessary resource for those who are working to save the lives of emergency victims. A communication system is beneficial to an EMS system only when it provides the operating personnel with the right kinds of communication at the right places at the right time.

In planning for the EMS communication system, and for every other EMS subsystem, there are two plans involved. The first is the areawide EMS plan, written by the EMS committee after an intensive survey of the area's emergency medical resources and identification of emergency medical needs. The committee developing this EMS plan must therefore include those able to identify these needs— physicians, hospital administrators, ambulance operators, and emergency medical technicians (EMTs)—and have available to it advice from someone knowledgeable in public-safety communications. These planners must reach decisions about the functions the communication system must perform at each step of the EMS sequence.

For such decisions, some familiarity with the capabilities and limitations of equipment and systems is necessary. These EMS committee planners will find this book of special value.

The second plan, a detailed communication plan based on the data in the overall EMS plan, is the province of someone with extensive experience and familiarity with public-safety communication equipment, licensing regulations, frequency problems, and system design and costs. This person will be responsible for determining precisely what items of equipment are needed at the dispatch center, in hospitals and ambulances, at relay stations, and at satellite receivers, and for drawing up detailed specifications against which purveyors can bid. Ideally this person should also be familiar with communication systems already in place in the area and in adjacent areas, and with the geographic and political constraints within which the system must function.

It is likely that much of this information will be available from the reports generated by the EMS committee. Some EMS committees are fortunate in having such a person as an able and willing member. Those less fortunate must bring in an outside expert. Many state communications offices have technical experts who can provide valuable assistance, together with a knowledge of coordination requirements, to local communications people. This combination of talents, where available, may provide the best solution.

Some systems have relied on expertise provided by a particular vendor. While this relieves local people of considerable work, it may have the disadvantages of providing less area expertise and of limiting the choice of equipment. Some have brought in a communications consultant—individual or firm—who has the advantages of extensive experience with EMS communication systems and a fresh and independent viewpoint, but with the disadvantage of unfamiliarity with local conditions. Against the consultant's fee, which may be substantial, should be set the potential savings a consultant's particular expertise should make possible.

To do the job well, a consultant will need not only the general EMS plan, but also a knowledge of the area's political, topographic, economic, and demographic characteristics. One purpose of this book, then, is to indicate the kinds of information an EMS committee must make available to the communications consultant.

The word *communication* means not only the technological transmission of information, as by telephone or radio, but also the exchange of information between people as a basis for mutual understanding. Both purposes are considered here, by providing EMS planners with a general knowledge of communications technology that can serve both as a tool in their EMS planning and as a bridge between physicians, hospital administrators, EMS providers, and the consumers concerned in the development of an EMS system. The arrangement of the chapters in the book provide the reader with the sequential steps in developing an effective EMS communication system. An important part of this developmental approach is the rationale provided for each step.

An effective evaluation of the present configuration and operational procedure of an EMS system is necessary in order to demonstrate the strengths and weaknesses of the system. This type of evaluation provides two important elements in developing an EMS communication system: (1) it establishes the communication requirements of the EMS system with its *present* configuration and operational procedures and (2) it establishes the communication requirements of the EMS system when the weaknesses of the EMS system are *corrected*, including necessary expansion. Through this technique, the design of the EMS communication system can effectively meet the present and future requirements of a specific EMS system. To the reader, this requirement may be all too obvious; however, it is the one of most neglected elements in an EMS communication system design. Communications, as a supporting resource, must be tailored to the specific operational procedure of a specific EMS system, as opposed to a package communication system where the EMS operational procedure must be modified to accommodate the capabilities of the available communication system.

Another of the most neglected elements in the design of an EMS communication system is the inclusion of tailored expansion capabilities. Again, to be effective, they must match the specific expansion program of the EMS system, in time schedules and equipment installation.

Chapter 1 places the communication system in proper perspective to the EMS system, that is as a supporting resource to an EMS plan of operation. The basic objective is the development of an EMS planning report. This report enables the communication support requirements to be readily identified and incorporated within the final EMS communication system design.

Chapter 2 identifies the elements of an EMS system and the considerations to be included in its development.

Chapter 3 provides guidance to the creation of an EMS council and its program objectives, including criteria for member selection, organization, responsibilities of the council committees, and types of data needed for preparing the EMS planning report.

Chapter 4 is concerned with the composition, evaluation, and coordination of an EMS planning report and with conducting the committee survey and sources of information, including available communications facilities.

Having established the EMS planning report and the criteria for the communications requirements that will support the existing and future EMS system, Chapter 5, provides an introduction to the later chapters on the development of an EMS communication system.

Chapter 6 concerns the various common functions an EMS communication system must provide, such as easy access by the public, response time, and applications of mobile and fixed station communication.

At this point, the EMS council may desire professional assistance. Chapter 7 introduces the services that may be provided by a communications consultant, including the techniques of interviewing prospective consultants, reviewing their proposals, and developing contractual arrangements.

Chapter 8 provides a nontechnical introduction to the design of an EMS communication system and thus-increases the capability to communicate with the consultant, or other technical personnel, on the planned system design, required capabilities, and techniques to achieve these ends.

Chapter 9 continues the nontechnical dialogue on the subject of developing the technical specifications for equipment procedures and vendor contract considerations. And Chapter 10 provides an overall summary of the book.

Frequently, the Federal Communications Commission (FCC) has promulgated regulations that may affect an EMS communication system design. Appendix A discusses the general functions of the Commission and selected regulations applicable to an EMS communication system.

A necessary adjunct to an EMS communication system is funding. Appendix B identifies some of the potential sources of funding by federal government agencies. Current information on their funding programs may be obtained by direct contact with the individual agency.

Following Appendix B is a section entitled Selected References and Resource Agencies. The reference material is arranged by subject matter and concludes with the name and address of selected federal agencies. Where the cost of the references is known, it is given. Others may or may not cost a modest fee.

Chapter 2

General Considerations

THE EMS SEQUENCE

There are essentially seven sequential functions involved in the operation of an emergency medical services system:

1. *Prevention:* Prevention involves both public education, in recognition of a medical emergency and in use of the EMS system, and such preventive measures as working for removal of highway hazards.
2. *Detection:* The EMS system can help in detection by such diverse means as public education in symptom recognition or by such diverse means as public education in symptom recognition or by providing highway users with the means of reporting a medical emergency.
3. *Notification:* The proper authorities must be notified that an emergency has occurred.
4. *Dispatch:* An appropriate vehicle must be dispatched as quickly as possible.
5. *On-Site Treatment:* On-the-scene emergency treatment, and extrication if necessary, leading to patient stabilization, must be provided by emergency medical technicians (EMTs) or paramedics.
6. *Transport:* Continuing care and supervision is necessary during transport of the patient to an appropriate medical facility.
7. *Emergency Department (ED) care:* The delivery of the patient to the ED transfers the responsibility for patient care to the receiving medical staff. However, in many EMS systems, the EMTs may provide temporary assistance in the ED.

In addition to the preceding steps, the following three steps complete the sequence of patient care and provide the historical record necessary for evaluating the ultimate impact of the EMS system on health care in the area:

8. *Acute In-Hospital Care:* After stabilizing emergency care, a patient with a substantial emergency medical problem would be transferred to the proper definitive care unit of the hospital.
9. *Recuperation:* Once the patient's condition has sufficiently improved, transfer to a general hospital ward or graded-care facility is in order.
10. *Rehabilitation:* The patient's return to family and employment.

RESOURCE MANAGEMENT

The rationale for organizing EMS on a regional basis is to provide more efficient management of emergency medical resources. Regional organization is established to ensure that minimum time is lost between the event creating the emergency and notification, that the nearest appropriate rescue vehicle is dispatched promptly, that the best possible emergency care is provided at the scene and in transit, and that the patient is taken to an emergency department that has been notified in advance and is capable of properly treating the patient.

The implications of effective resource management are tremendous. It requires, at the outset, a degree of cooperation between public service agencies—police, fire, civil defense, and the central EMS; between political jurisdictions—towns, cities, and counties; and between private service providers—ambulance companies, hospitals, and telephone companies. To most regions this is a new idea. Each of these entities has its own autonomy, often jealously guarded. Some measure of this autonomy must be yielded in the interest of public good and patient welfare if an EMS system is to work. More than one burgeoning EMS system has foundered on the territorial imperatives of its constituent organizations.

These often-conflicting interests can be reconciled only if everyone is in the act from the start. The primary function of an EMS committee, during its early deliberations, may well be to serve as a sounding board for special interests—as a place where differences and concerns can be identified and dealt with and where all can participate in developing the area EMS plan. The composition of an EMS committee is discussed below.

The efficiency of EMS system resource management in an area

will be proportional to the authority, based on political acceptance, of the EMS management organization. Where counties are politically strong, the county government may be the best organization to manage the system. Elsewhere, a separate corporation, or a hospital consortium, or a municipal public-safety department may afford the most viable system management. The primary job of one EMS subcommittee should be to determine what feasible form of management organization will have the authority to make its decisions stick.

PUBLIC EDUCATION

Public education for EMS is too often thought of only in terms of telephone stickers to be distributed after a single EMS number has been agreed to. In fact, public education should be one of the initial concerns of an EMS committee. Educating the public in the concept that EMS, like police and fire, is an essential community service, is crucial.

Ultimately an EMS system must rely on the political entities of the area both for the effectiveness of system operations and for the necessary financing. Local governments are more likely to assume these responsibilities when it is clear to them that this is what the public demands. Committee members should seek opportunities to address civic groups, town meetings, and legislatures on the nature and importance of an emergency medical services system. Active involvement of people from the news media in the public education subcommittee can be invaluable.

Public education may also include lay training in recognition of symptoms and first aid of victims of medical emergencies and, once the system is in operation, in the use of the EMS system. (See Appendix C, Selected References and Resource Agencies.)

TRAINING

Any system for emergency care is only as good as those who administer such care—the physicians, emergency nurses, paramedics, and EMTs. It is thus appropriate that EMT, professional-refresher, and public first-aid training has been the area of greatest initial emphasis and has made the most notable progress among EMS systems. The level of requirements for ambulance-hospital communication are directly proportional to the level of EMT training: the higher the skills of the EMT at the scene of an emergency, the greater is his or her need for professional medical advice. This is true because most of the advanced life-support techniques, such as defibrillation, intubation, and administration of intravenous fluids—invasive medical techniques—usually cannot be performed by paramedics or EMTs without specific authorization or direction by a physician. Where this constraint is not written into state laws, it is usually enforced by local medical practice.

Similarly, the question, which inevitably arises, of whether to treat at the scene or to transport immediately to a hospital may be relatively simple for an ambulance attendant whose skills are largely in bandaging and splinting. But for the paramedic, who has the ability to perform more advanced life-saving techniques, the choice is likely to be more difficult, requiring the advice of a physician.

The training of volunteers as EMTs and paramedics may be difficult, particularly in rural areas, because of the time and personal expense required for training. Further, rural volunteers may get insufficient practice to ensure skill maintenance. Yet it is these rural areas, where ambulance runs are often long, that have the greatest need for sophisticated pre-hospital care and communications. An EMS system that can underwrite the training of these volunteers, equip their vehicles with the necessary medical and communication gear, and provide squad members with tours of urban EMS or hospital duty, can go far toward alleviating this problem.

In many areas (and in some states as required by law), fire and police personnel, who are often the first on the scene of a medical emergency, are trained in Advanced First Aid or as basic EMTs. Such training can contribute not only to the saving of lives but also to furthering cooperation among the three emergency response agencies.

Another area of training, of course, must be in the operation and care of radio equipment. Some EMS projects have conducted courses of such training for EMTs and for emergency care nurses and physicians. Projects that have not made such training a part of their program sometimes report a reluctance of emergency department (ED) personnel to use the equipment, or a tendency to leave it turned down. As shown later in Chapter 4, where ambulance communications with the hospital are relayed by landline from the central resource communications center (RCC), this particular problem is obviated for ED personnel. On the other hand, if the telephone line becomes disabled, a hospital without a backup radio can be devoid of emergency communications.

In the conduct of EMT training programs, ideally by physicians who will subsequently be working with the EMTs, it is desirable to have an EMS radio monitor in the classroom to give the students a feel for system operation and to tape record situations for problem-solving exercises.

MEDICAL DIRECTION

Because the EMS is to be a system for emergency medical care, physician input and professional medical control is essential. This should mean many things: overall medical supervision and monitoring of the system operation to ensure that the emergency medical needs of the area are being properly met; provision of emergency care advice to the caller; supervision and integration into the system of such auxiliary medical services as the poison-control and drug-abuse centers; and physician supervision of and participation in EMT and paramedic training.

A primary role of professional medical direction is the supervision of and responsibility for the actions of the nurses and emergency medical technicians providing emergency care. In most states only a physician may assume this responsibility. Basic life-support measures, usually considered as first aid, do not always legally require strict medical supervision, but when advanced life-support is required, physician supervision becomes mandatory [55]. Usually this is provided by radio communication between the physician at a central area hospital and the emergency medical technician at the scene. In urban areas, to avoid accidental mid-direction resulting from multiple users of a doctor-talk channel, it is essential to regionalize medical supervision by designating a primary hospital center for this purpose.

FINANCING

The EMS council from the start must seek ways of financing the planning, management, and operation of the system. Recently, various federal, state, local, and private resources have been available to help with start-up costs (see Appendix B), but it is clear that an EMS system must eventually be supported by the area it serves—whether through taxes, fees for service, subscriptions, cost-sharing, voluntary contributions, or some combination of these. Such support will become possible when, as a result of public education, EMS is recognized—together with the police and fire services—as an essential public-safety function.

A natural tendency in new EMS systems, with outside start-up funds, is to defer solication of public support until the system has been put into operation, on the assumption that government officials and the public will be unwilling to allow an essential public service to lapse. This is a gamble, but one that can at least be hedged by obtaining prior commitments for future system funding once the system has been shown to be successful. A detailed economic study comparing the projected cost—to the citizen and to local governments—of the EMS system, as opposed to that of the fragmented care previously available, may prove persuasive.

Funding for development of telecommunication systems within states, regions, or local jurisdictions is, in general, single-function oriented. For example, education funds must be wholly spent for the activities of an education system; rural agriculture data and contact systems utilized for agriculture only; law-enforcement funds for enforcement systems activities; medical service funds for medical services; and so on.

The establishment of the Federal Inter-Agency EMS Committee under the 1973 EMS Act appeared to encourage cost-sharing of community and regional telecommunication systems. But, most federal support available for development of telecommunication systems or operating services remain single-function oriented. There is still not available, in one package, federal assistance for the development of a total emergency services telecommunication system that can meet single agency needs on a joint-use basis, which would thereby effect savings. Consequently the present federal funding sources encourage local governments to proliferate the development of independent systems, which are generally uneconomical. It therefore remains a clear responsibility of local and regional developers and EMS councils to bring together available funds and establish an acceptable formula for cost-sharing support of EMS telecommunications (see Appendix B).

INTERAGENCY COORDINATION

As already indicated, an EMS system requires close cooperation between all emergency response agencies. Ideally this cooperation will take the form of a 911 public-safety answering point (PASP), and a central resource control center (RCC), shared by police, fire, and EMS. Where this is done, the public is assured the most direct access, and also that the most prompt and appropriate response to any emergency will occur. Collocation in a single dispatch center—while economical and functionally desirable—is not essential; the PSAP may be tied by dedicated telephone lines directly to the three (EMS, Police, and Fire) geographically separate dispatch centers. Even in systems where a central medical emergency dispatcher

(CMED) is reached by a special medical emergency number, direct contact and close cooperation with the police, fire, and other emergency response services is essential. Regardless of how well the medical number has been publicized, some emergency medical calls will continue to come to police and fire and to telephone operators, who must be able to transfer these calls directly to the CMED. Also, police and fire personnel are often the first to have knowledge of a medical emergency. Conversely, the CMED must be able to call instantly for assistance from the police and fire departments, when appropriate.

Such cooperation, like that among cities and counties, may not be easy to achieve. But involvement of fire and police chiefs in EMS planning may lead to the realization that the efficiency of their departments, as well as their public image, would be best served by full cooperation with and participation in an EMS system.

REGIONALIZATION

To date, no pat formula has evolved for defining an EMS region. Definition by hospital catchment area may ignore political obstacles to cooperation; conversely, definition by political boundaries—or, more recently, by Health Services Area (HSA) boundaries—may ignore patient flow patterns and result in needless duplication of services. Definition by hospital services, requiring that an EMS system include within its geographic boundaries all necessary medical services, could result in unwieldy size [4].

It may be more fruitful to define a region in terms of *regional goals.* The EMS system should make the area's medical resources more available to the citizenry; it should improve the quality of emergency care; and it should organize and efficiently manage the available emergency medical resources. The region, then, will be that area in which, given the local political, geographic, and socioeconomic realities, these goals can be substantially achieved.

The local realities are not unalterable, however, and should not be built permanently into the system design. Political differences can be reconciled; geographic obstacles may yield to advanced forms of transportation and communications; and EMS economics, properly understood, may dictate the expansion, rather than the limitation, of an EMS system. An optimal EMS system, then, may be one in which the reach is greater than the grasp, in which the overall planning will allow for, and prepare the ground for, ultimate expansion, while providing for full system implementation within an area where it is presently feasible.

PLANNING FOR EXPANSION

A phenomenal growth of EMS systems has taken place in recent years, both in the establishment of new systems and in the expansion of those already started. This process becomes inevitable as more people learn of the benefits of systematized emergency care, and desirable in the extension of such care to previously unserved areas and in the inclusion of a greater breadth of medical resources. Federal planning envisions a time when the country will be covered by a network of contiguous interconnecting EMS systems.

Thus, while initial planning of an EMS project will reflect chiefly the needs of a particular community or area, it should also allow for future expansion to adjacent areas not yet served by EMS, for coordination with neighboring EMS systems, and for eventual participation in a statewide or interstate EMS system.

In practical terms this means, for instance, that—in an EMS system adjacent to unserved areas—the EMS resource communications center (RCC) should be designed modularly, with the floor space, structural strength, and so on to accommodate the equipment and personnel that would be needed to serve an expanded system. Antenna heights and locations should not be solely determined by local requirements.

No EMS system is an island unto itself: radio waves do not stop at county lines, and disasters do not respect service jurisdictions. For these reasons it is essential that an EMS system cooperate and coordinate with adjacent EMS systems, both for frequency coordination to prevent interference (or worse, misdirection) and to ensure availability, when needed, of mutual aid. These considerations will also affect antenna location and design, transmitter power, and frequency allocation; and will require direct communication links between the RCCs of neighboring systems.

The seven sequential functions involved in the operation of an EMS system are the actions required of the public and service agencies that together comprise the EMS system. The effectiveness of the system is directly proportional to that of the resource management when applied to the many parts that make the system functional as an integrated unit. With this identification of the parameters of an EMS system, the need is for an action group to be responsible for the evaluation and development of the EMS programs used by the emergency service agencies and the public. The next chapter identifies the EMS council as the logical vehicle to direct the development of an EMS plan of operation.

II. Finance.
  A. Subcommittees.
    1. Funding of EMS council work.
    2. Sources of funding for EMS system.
    3. Costs of equipment, salaries, maintenance, and so on.
III. Law.
  A. Subcommittees.
    1. Laws relating to EMS council and EMS system operation.
    2. Laws governing providers.
      a. Standards for ambulances, equipment, EMTs.
      b. Legal protection: mutual aid, good samaritan.
      c. Payment—insurance, medicare, fees for service, cost-sharing.
      d. Communications: local and state regulations; FCC rules.
IV. Medical Survey.
  A. Subcommittees.
    1. EMS resources.
      a. Ambulances and rescue squads: equipment, EMT training, access and control, links with hospitals; kinds of squads.
      b. Hospitals and emergency departments: range of services offered; 24-hour availability; categorization; communications.
      c. Evaluation—availability of data base.
      d. Consultation expertise available.
    2. EMS needs and priorities: kinds of medical emergencies; where they occur; alternative ways of meeting the needs.
V. Prior EMS Planning.
  A. What EMS system or EMS communications planning has already been done at state or local levels? What disaster planning? What communication nets (such as civil defense) are in operation?
VI. Geography and Demography.
  A. What should the EMS area consist of? Are county lines the determining factor? What is the catchment area of the hospitals? What is the distribution, composition, characteristics of the population? Does topography pose special problems in transportation or communications? Are any areas, or population segments, denied access to emergency medical care? What precedents are there for cooperation among the area's political jurisdictions, public service organizations, and so on?

For further information see Appendix C references [1]-[6].

Once the reports are in from these committees and have been thoroughly discussed, an executive group of committee chairpersons can begin drafting the EMS plan. This plan should represent a consensus of the EMS council members on what the needs and problems of the area are, and how, in general terms, these should be addressed. This may require a restructuring within the council, establishing separate committees to prepare sections of the EMS plan dealing with communications, training, public education, categorization, evaluation, administration, transportation, referral protocols, financing, and whatever else is judged necessary.

The elements of an EMS system have now been identified and an EMS council has been activated to investigate and evaluate the effectiveness of existing agencies and programs and to develop needed improvements. Chapter 4 develops the EMS planning report that documents the findings of the committee members and the decisions of the council.

Chapter 4

The EMS Planning Report

An EMS planning report includes the community and area EMS goals, planning data analysis, and a plan of action to achieve specified objectives. The report provides the members of the EMS council and agencies having EMS responsibilities with a compilation of data that represents their collective decisions on matters of EMS program objectives for the community and the area, and the means to be used in their fulfillment.

The planning report documents the results of the council planning in three areas of the EMS:

1. The kinds of EMS programs and supporting resources needed in the area to provide the degree of excellence desired by the council members and the supporting agencies.
2. An inventory and analysis of the present community programs and supporting resources.
3. By comparing items 1 and 2 above, it identifies the additional required resources and operational arrangements.

The data to be gathered by the council during their fact-finding interviews and the on-site investigations will be used to evaluate the status of the available EMS programs and pertinent resources of the participating agencies.

The planning report identifies the discrepancies between the first part of the report—the *required*—with the second part of the report— the *available*—and identifies the *needs* of the EMS programs and the supporting resources to achieve the desired objectives. This is the planning report formula as detailed in succeeding paragraphs. The next step is to determine the kinds of corrective actions required, where they are needed, the mechanics of change, and a schedule for compliance.

PLANNING REPORT FORMULA

What is Required: (The total area EMS programs, services, and resources required in the EMS system as determined by the EMS council members and supporting agencies.)

Minus

What is Available: (The existing EMS programs and resources that are operational and can be utilized to meet the EMS system plan requirements.)

Equals

What is Needed: (The EMS programs that must be developed, and resources (service, personnel and materials) that must be provided in the area to achieve the results desired.)

COMPOSITION OF THE PLANNING REPORT

A planning report should communicate to the users and supporters of the EMS system the present status of the supporting communication system, recommended changes, what they will accomplish, and a program for accomplishment. It should also provide the consultant with the information needed to design an EMS radio communication system.

The implementation schedule in the planning report should coordinate related program elements in a phased approach. For instance, if the EMS program provides for the development of a biomedical telemetry system, this should be timed with the development of the hospital EMS program that would provide the biomedical equipment and trained personnel. The development of the public safety answering point (PSAP) is time-phased with the activation of the common, multidigit or 911 emergency telephone number. The colocation of the central EMS communications in the emergency services resources communication center (RCC) is time-phased with EMS program requirements and development of the EMS communication system. In turn, the development of the EMS communication system is time-phased with supporting activities such as funding, deliveries, construction, trained personnel, FCC licensing, and so on. This process continues so that as the EMS programs progress, the supporting communications are developed on a time-phased schedule.

DEFINING EMS NEEDS

An EMS program is basically a plan of action to be carried out by the catchment area emergency medical service agencies in response to a given medical emergency. The number and type of emergencies will determine the size and complexity of the program to be developed. Some actions are confined to the services of the EMS vehicles and receiving hospitals. Others will include additional public-safety agencies such as the police and fire departments, in a support role.

EMS needs can be defined in terms of: (1) the kinds of medical emergencies to which a response is necessary; (2) the types of responses required; and (3) the sequence of EMS operations.

Identification of the kinds of emergencies to which the EMS system must respond may entail consideration of natural disasters, such as floods or tornados, to which the area is vulnerable. Industries in a community may present health hazards that require advance planning in an EMS program. A major highway in the community may be a source of vehicular accidents. There may be seasonal medical emergencies from such public activities as swimming, boating, mountain climbing, skiing, snowmobiles, and the like. The local airport may present hazards requiring special EMS programs. This composite of demands represents the problem to be solved by the EMS program.

Identification of the types of EMS resources required for adequate response may lead to the conclusion that several vehicles and EMTs providing basic life support are required, with a lesser number of vehicles at the advanced level for carrying paramedics and the multiplicity of equipment and drugs needed for advanced emergency medical care. Additionally, during a disaster response there may be requirements for traffic controls, alerting and staffing of all hospital emergency rooms, assignment of physicians at the scene for emergency treatment and medication, setting up emergency hospital beds and additional medical equipment, using the resources of area hospitals, requesting the state for National Guard assistance with helicopters, ambulances, and medical personnel.

The EMS program should detail the sequence of the reactions to be taken by the medical personnel in responding to a medical emergency. This starts with citizen awareness of the emergency, the call for assistance to the public-safety communication center, and the interconnection to the emergency medical service communication center. The reaction by the dispatcher and subsequent reactions by the members of the EMS system and supporting resource agencies will depend upon the nature and type of the medical emergency and the availability of communications, personnel, equipment, and related resources.

In assessing EMS needs, data for a specific time period should be gathered on the following:

1. The total number of patients who required emergency care in the hospital emergency department.
2. The total number of patients who needed EMS vehicle transport service.
3. The number, by type, of emergency medical needs treated—heart attack, acute illness, traumatic injury, poison, and so on.
4. The total number of emergencies answered—by day of week and time of day.
5. The total number of patients who, having called for EMS, died before reaching the hospital.
6. The response times of the current system.

EMS COMMITTEE SURVEY

In establishing the program, the EMS council should survey existing emergency-care resources. The survey at each component should be by a team representing the component being surveyed and those depending on it for support.

A survey of the current status of the community EMS (1) training for medical treatment at the scene; (2) EMS communications; (3) emergency medical transportation; and (4) emergency hospital facilities. The following kinds of questions should be asked.

Training for Medical Treatment at the Scene: Is training in emergency care available to the first responder? Is such training available through industrial safety programs, school curriculum, or adult education programs? How many students complete these courses? What emergency medical training is required for police and fire department personnel? Are they tested periodically for skill retention? What training is required of EMS vehicle attendants—first aid, advanced first aid, EMT, EMT-paramedic? Of the total number of these personnel, how many have the required emergency medical training? Are they tested periodically for skill retention?

Emergency Medical Service Communications: What are the means of communications available to the citizen requiring EMS? If the telephone number 911 is provided, how often is it used in comparison with other emergency telephone numbers? Can the present emergency communication system provide 24-hour service for two-way communication between hospitals, emergency medical vehicles, police and fire departments, and other agencies involved in EMS? Is there a resource communications center (RCC) that receives all EMS calls? Does this RCC dispatch emergency vehicles and personnel, or transfer the call to the agency that does the dispatching? Does the dispatcher have CMED training? Can the emergency communication facilities function as an integrated EMS system? Is all of the communication equipment operational? What is the communication-equipment maintenance program? Is it effective? Are there operational stand-by electrical power plants for the communication center and remote equipment sites? Are there stand-by trained dispatchers? Does the RCC maintain current and relevant records on vehicle and personnel dispatch, response and arrival time, and turnaround time?

Emergency Medical Transportation: Do the EMS emergency vehicles meet the standards specified by the American College of Surgeons, the National Research Council, and appropriate Department of Transportation specifications? What is the operational condition of the present equipment? How many EMS vehicle attendants trained as EMTs are available for each vehicle dispatched to the scene of a medical emergency? How many EMS vehicles are available full time and part time; what are their stand-by locations; are they accessible to various geographic areas? Have all drivers of EMS emergency vehicles completed the defensive driving training course as prescribed by the National Safety Council? Do the EMS vehicle attendants provide medical records on the victim's condition, treatments rendered, and the effects?

Emergency Hospital Facilities: Has an evaluation of the hospital emergency department been completed that includes both the adequacy of the facilities and the availability and training of the staff? Are there procedures for segregating urgent from nonurgent patients, and are methods used to maintain the emergency department for urgent patients? Are centers for poison-control care, psychiatric care, and drug-abuse medical care available? Are medical records adequate and available to the staff? Are protocols established for hospital assignment and transfer of patients?

The preceding areas of investigation are not all-inclusive, nor do they fully probe the subjects of EMS. They only identify some of the critical areas that the EMS council members should investigate and personally observe to understand the magnitude of the problem areas.

This survey of the catchment area emergency medical care resources is essential to the development of the EMS plan for an effective system in the geographic area, and for compatibility with adjacent EMS service area systems. Its importance should be apparent to the EMS council members, because it will be the adequacy of their own services and facilities that the council members will be reviewing.

Response to a Medical Emergency

Table 4-1 outlines the sequence of actions and reactions by personnel responding to a medical emergency call from a citizen. When an existing EMS program is evaluated in this manner, the sufficiencies and deficiencies become apparent. The response time, adequacy of communications, availability of personnel and equipment, response of supporting agencies, and qualifications of personnel are some of the items for evaluation. Corrective action may then be developed to improve the EMS program. The list of survey items is only illustrative. Each council must develop its own requirements.

To be realistic, the evaluation should be of services actually being provided, and may take several months. This fact-finding EMS program evaluation is not a one-shot operation, but a continuing activity. By revaluing at regular intervals, defects in the service can be identified and remedial action initiated.

The EMS council should schedule meeting for the review and recording of the committee reports. These reviews and progress reports provide an opportunity to evaluate the scope of the survey and make desirable adjustments, and also serve as a stimulus to the agencies involved to upgrade the emergency medical services system. They also serve the important function of providing a forum at which disagreements can be aired and reconciled, and complaints can be answered.

The Communications Inventory

When the system design includes the possible utilization of existing EMS system communications, a complete inventory is required to determine what communication facilities are in operation and where they are located. An example of a communication inventory form is shown as Table 4-2.

Table 4-1. Sequential Responses to a Medical Emergency

Action Required	Results Required	Responsible Agent	Needed Resources	Available Resources
Answer call for EMS	Evaluate caller's needs for medical care and response.	CMED	A 911 or equal emergency medical communications centers, cotenant with other public safety communication centers, and staffed with CMEDs.	The actual situation in the catchment area, as shown by the survey of EMS programs, will be recorded in this column.
Immediate medical care	Provide immediate response to the medical emergency. Dispatch EMS vehicle and EMTs to the scene of the medical emergency.	CMED and the emergency medical vehicle service.	Medically equipped vehicle, EMTs, communications with the CMED, EMTs and the medical consultant.	
Same as above.	Diagnosis of medical emergency at the scene by EMTs, and advise CMED.	Same as above.	Same as above	
Same as above.	Selection of hospital. Advise hospital and establish communication between the EMT and the receiving hospital emergency department.	Same as above	Same as above, plus the receiving hospital.	

Table 4–1. (continued)

Action Required	Results Required	Responsible Agent	Needed Resources	Available Resources
Prepare patient for transport to the hospital.	Communication between the EMTs and the medical consultant.	Emergency medical vehicle service and the medical consultant	Communications between the EMTs and the medical consultant.	The actual situation in the community, as shown by the survey of EMS programs, will be recorded in this column.
Same as above.	If necessary, transmission of patients vital signs from the scene of the emergency to the medical consultant for observation and diagnosis.	Same as above.	Same as above, plus possible telemetry.	
Same as above.	Direction and supervision of the EMTs by the medical consultant for treatment and medication necessary to stabilize the patient.	Same as above.	Same as above.	
Transport of patient to the hospital.	Maintain voice and telemetry communications between the medical consultant and the EMTs for continued emergency care of the patient during transport to the receiving hospital.	Same as above.	Same as above.	

Table 4–1. (continued)

				The actual situation in the community, as shown by the survey of EMS programs, will be recorded in this column.
Delivery of the patient to the receiving hospital emergency department.	The patient medical records of the diagnosis, treatment, and medication provided by the EMTs are delivered to the physician at the receiving hospital.	Emergency medical vehicle service and the receiving hospital physician.	Appropriate hospital facility, with a medical staff having pre-delivery knowledge of the medical emergency.	
Continuing emergency medical care.	Immediate medical care of the patient to further stabilize the patient preparatory to transfer to an appropriate care unit of the receiving hospital.	Hospital emergency department.	Medical staff, equipment, and supplies for necessary emergency care, and communication facilities within the hospital.	

Table 4-2. Communication Inventory

Licensee: FCC Licensed Service: Date:

A	B	C	D	E	F	G
System Elements and Locations	*Operational Frequencies*	*Trans. Power (watts)*	*Mode of Operation*	*Interconnect Locations*	*Using Agencies*	*Assigned Functions*
Base Station Bravo-Model T, purchased 1955. Loving Arms Hospital	T–155.340 R–155.340	100	FM	Mobiles	Ever Ready Ambulance	EMS
Mobile Transceiver Cargo Model X, purchased 1955. Ever Ready Ambulance Service	T–155.340 R–155.340	30	FM	Base Station	Loving Arms Hospital	EMS in Coyote County
Remote-located Base Station Aider Model PP, purchased 1956. High Point Hill	T–155.340 R–155.340	60	FM	Mobile Base Station	Loving Arms Hospital Ever Ready Ambulance Service	Remote-located base station

Note: This is a hypothetical example for illustration only.

Once the accounting has been accomplished, an evaluation is made of each item to determine its usability in the new system. The evaluation should:

1. Confirm the need for the item in the existing or new system application.
2. Evaluate, if it is to be retained, the mechanical and electronic condition of the item, and determine the cost of bringing the item to maximum performance.
3. Review the maintenance record of the item to evaluate the reliability and determine the maintenance cost factor by extrapolation over a 1-, 3-, and 5-year period.
4. If required, determine the one-time costs to modify the item for a specific use in the new system.
5. Total the one-time and recurring costs for 1-, 3-, and 5-year periods, and compare the same criteria with the procurement and maintenance costs of the new item.
6. Establish the economical point of diminishing returns to determine whether it is more economical to repair or replace the item (when the repair cost is 50 percent or more of the replacement cost).

The Resource Communication Center (RCC)

The community or area being surveyed by the EMS council may have one or more RCCs serving the present needs of the public-safety agencies. Members of the council should be aware of the location of these centers, which may be presently at police and fire stations, EMS vehicle services, or receiving hospitals that operate ambulances. The agency administrators and RCC directors have information on the services they provide and the merits and weaknesses of each. Discussions with the people using the services of the RCC may disclose additional data on the ability of the center to provide the EMS communications required for their needs.

These RCCs may have one of several configurations:

Configuration 1. The center may receive all emergency telephone calls, and provide dispatch service for all medical, police, fire, and utility agencies.

Configuration 2. The center may receive emergency telephone calls for police and fire departments, dispatch the police and fire vehicles, and relay requests for emergency medical service to the EMS vehicle station or receiving hospital, or to a CMED.

Configuration 3. There may be a separate telephone number and communication center for each public-safety agency, including the emergency medical vehicle services and the receiving hospital.

In planning for a single EMS dispatch center, the EMS council will need to consider the following attributes of these three configurations (see Table 4-3).

Configuration 1. The first configuration requires the communication center to be located in a secure area, separate from any of the public-safety agencies being served. It should be staffed 24 hours each day by CMEDs for the EMS system, dispatchers for the police and fire departments, and operators of the emergency telephone number 911 PSAP.

Emergency telephone numbers from the public should be received on the emergency number 911, or the multidigit number used by the area or for each public-safety agency. These calls should be received by operators trained in the techniques of obtaining, in a minimum of time, pertinent information from callers that are under duress, and making immediate response to their needs.

The response may take any of several forms. Depending on the caller's needs, the call should be immediately interconnected to the appropriate dispatcher for reply and reaction. The 911 operator originally receiving the call should remain on the line long enough to determine if the call has been appropriately transferred.

The RCC should have both radio and telephone communications to the critical areas of each public-safety agency, for the CMED, to the attendants of the emergency medical vehicle service, the poison center, emergency departments, and appropriate medical control facilities. This dispatcher should also monitor radio calls between the ambulances and the hospitals. Depending on the regional requirements for sophistication, the resources available to the CMED to assist in expediting a response to an emergency call would include:

a. A computerized data bank from which readouts are displayed. A small keyboard is used by the dispatcher to obtain data such as availability of an EMS vehicle, availability of hospital facilities, road conditions, pertinent telephone numbers, assigned radio channels, and similar data related to the emergency and the needed response.
b. Rear-view screen projections of sectional maps showing the area in which the emergency occurred, with details of nearest hospital and emergency medical vehicle service locations, and other public safety services.

c. Radio and telephone communications with adjoining community communication centers, used to coordinate responses to emergencies that cross community boundary lines. In the event of major emergencies, or a single disaster requiring facilities and services beyond the response capabilities of these communities, this emergency communication center should be capable of requesting and coordinating emergency medical services support from neighboring jurisdictions and state agencies.

In summary, this first type of communication center has the personnel, training, facilities, and resources required to respond, with judgment and timeliness, to calls from the public and public-safety agencies for emergency medical services.

Configuration 2. The second configuration of a communication center is usually associated with a police department, because they normally have more emergency calls than the other public-safety agencies. The center may be located within the agency facilities, or in a separate location with interconnecting communication channels to the agencies being served. When appropriate, the Civil Defense agency's emergency operating center (EOC) may accommodate the communications center for the community public-safety agencies.

Calls to this type of center for the emergency medical service may be in three categories: (1) requests for an ambulance; (2) requests for the poison center; and (3) all others. The dispatcher may transfer the call or relay a message to the emergency medical vehicle service. Calls for the poison center are transferred to that center. All other calls are transferred to the attendant at the hospital emergency department.

This type of center is normally staffed with police-oriented personnel. There is minimal, if any, training in functions of the other public-safety agencies. The public has the advantage of calling a single emergency number, but may not receive the expeditious and trained handling of a medical emergency that would be received by the first type of communications center.

Configuration 3: The third type is not a center; it is virtually three or more centers, one for each emergency public-safety agency service—the emergency medical vehicle service, hospital, poison center, police department, fire department, and utility service.

The public must dial the separate multidigit number of the public safety agency that the caller *believes* can react to the emergency being reported. There can be delays in obtaining the telephone

Table 4-3. Summary of Typical Communication Centers

PROGRAM	General Objectives	SUPPORTING COMMUNICATION
		Provide an EMS communication system that will enable every citizen to receive an immediate response to an emergency medical call with timely and proficient medical service.
Bringing together various aspects of emergency medical services operated by different geographic and institutional jurisdictions with new and more satisfactory operational and administrative arrangements.	Configuration 1	
Central and immediate citizen access to the emergency medical system.	A qualified central medical emergency dispatcher (CMED) who efficiently coordinates and manages the EMS resources.	A coordinated, integrated EMS communications center that provides the communication links between the EMS system dispatch centers, other communication centers, hospitals, rescue and emergency medical care vehicle, and the functional integration with police and fire departments and civil defense.
Training of citizens in the effective use of the emergency medical response system		Establish communication from the medical control center and its supporting hospital facilities in the RCC.
Provide an emergency medical care system that will enable every citizen to receive an immediate response to an emergency call and receive timely and efficient emergency medical service.		Provide the medical catchment area with the telephone system 911 (common) emergency number and auxiliary services of dial-tone-first, hold and re-ring, and forcible disconnect.
Establish an appropriate medical control center.		A hospital emergency department communication system that includes radio voice and, where appropriate, telemetry, with the emergency medical vehicle service, dedicated telephone service for intra- and inter-hospital communications, and radio and telephone communication with the central emergency medical dispatcher(CMED).
Cooperating receiving hospital emergency department staffed 24 hours with physicians, nurses, and related personnel. Equipped with a state-of-the-art medical equipment, supplies, and communication facilities necessary to provide adequate emergency medical service.		

Table 4-3 (continued)

An emergency medical vehicle service with EMTs on 24-hour alert. Emergency medical vehicles equipped with adequate life-support equipment for on-the-scene diagnosis, emergency treatment, and medication.	Emergency medical vehicle service with mobile multi-channel radio communication for voice and, where appropriate, telemetry.
Training of CMEDs and other personnel, including EMTs, paramedics, emergency physicians, and nurses.	Methods for on-line monitoring of appropriate communication channels for classroom examples. Recordings of specific examples for classroom study. Laboratory set-up for training in equipment operation and simulated experience. Assessment of realistic emergency situation handling, in the laboratory, similar to aircraft controller simulated experience training. Continued observation and audit of proficiency and performance throughout work experiences.
Develop computer-controlled EMS data retrieval system.	Computer EMS data file material is made available to the CMED by visual presentation. Tape recordings of the callers and dispatchers conversations plus date and time of occurrences.
	Configuration 2
The utilization of existing public-safety communication facilities to include emergency medical service.	The police department communication center may be designated as the receiving agency for all public calls for emergency medical service.

Table 4-3. (continued)

PROGRAM	General Objectives	SUPPORTING COMMUNICATION
		Configuration 2
Establishment of a multidigit number the public can use to report a medical emergency and request service. The agency receiving the call determines the reacting agency.		Calls for EMS service or information are transferred or relayed to the emergency medical vehicle service, or to an emergency medical department. Dispatchers may have access to police and fire department radio communication systems to request EMS support. Radio communication with the state law-enforcement agency may be by cross-monitoring. In many cases, coordination by dedicated telephone lines is preferable.
EMTs are called from a duty roster. The hospital provides 24-hour switchboard service for hospital-oriented service systems.		EMTs are on standby to receive calls by telephone or public-safety radio communications. EMS is a secondary or subsidiary service to an existing public safety agency.
		Configuration 3
The citizen uses the telephone for direct contact to a hospital, emergency vehicle service, police department, or fire department for emergency medical service.		The citizen selects the multidigit number from the telephone directory, operator, or other information source for the agency needed to respond to the medical emergency.
		The agency called uses their communication facilities to respond or relay the request to another agency for response and support.
		Responsibility is difficult to document. EMS is a subsidiary service among public-safety agencies.

number to dial, whatever reference is used. Another choice is to dial "0" on the telephone, advise the operator of the emergency public-safety agency wanted, and either receive a number to dial, or if no other exchange is involved, the operator may dial the number for the caller. Either way, there is a loss of time compared to the use of the emergency telephone number 911 that everyone can memorize.

The use of the multidigit number of a specific public agency can result in further delay in reaching the desired agency if the caller must be referred to another agency for necessary action. In many configurations of this type, the EMS response is usually reduced to a telephone switchboard operator at a hospital, receiving calls for an ambulance service or the alerting of the emergency room staff.

In summary, EMS is, to an extent, served by the communications of configuration 3, but this option does not contain the time-saving elements needed by the emergency medical system to satisfy an urgent need for action.

The configuration of the three communication systems identified in the preceding paragraphs and in Table 4-3, and their variations, are the first points of investigation by the EMS council to identify and evaluate the existing and available communication systems in the community.

COORDINATION

When the planning report is completed, it should be endorsed by all agencies involved in the EMS system showing their agreement with the programs and with the proposed actions to make them effective. The planning report should also indicate the need for any funding from government or private sources and, if required, the need for any legislative action.

Federal Grants

The data in the planning report can also be used in applications to federal agencies for grants to be used in developing an EMS communication system. The U.S. Department of Health, Education and Welfare has issued publication number (HSA) 75-2013, February 1975, entitled *Program Guidelines for EMS Systems.* [4] The introduction of this publication states in part:

This policy statement is intended to help applicants understand the legislation, regulations, guidelines and related administrative procedures. It also familiarizes the applicant with the application procedures, and post-award project administration.

The publication also includes "Application Factors" used by the agency in evaluating requests for grants. Under a subheading of "Communications," there are ten questions that are applicable to the development of the EMS planning report:

1. Does the applicant describe the communication system to include a 911 access, central dispatch, medical consultation, linkages between ambulances, EMTs, hospitals, and other public-safety personnel?
2. Does the communication system support the medical requirements of the EMS system? Does the system consider linkages appropriate for disaster situations?
3. Does the application indicate that adequate engineering has been completed or is planned for the total communications system?
4. Does the communication system include education and training programs for use by all personnel involved?
5. Does the communication system plan address the community emergency needs for voice and telemetry?
6. Does the system include provision for command control during the medical consultation mode?
7. Has consideration been given to communication interfaces with such innovative programs as Military Assistance to Safety in Traffic programs (MAST) and medical air evacuation capabilities?
8. Does the communication component consider the public education program associated with access usage of the EMS communication system?
9. Is there an operations protocol [manual] to be developed for system users?
10. Has the licensure issue(s) been addressed and/or worked out?

There are similar publications from other federal agencies that are useful in evaluating the completeness of the EMS planning report. See the Selected References and Resource Agencies at the end of this book for recommended reading.

In the final analysis, the planning report, which is developed in four parts, concerns the community or area EMS programs and the supporting communication system. *The first part* identifies the desired degree of excellence in each of the EMS programs. *The second part* identifies the present status of, or the lack of, these programs and the supporting communications. *The third part* identifies what must be accomplished to achieve the desired degree of excellence in the programs and the communication system. *The fourth part* details how these plans are to be accomplished.

The planning report thus becomes the master plan for the development of the EMS system and the supporting communication components. When it is developed in phases over an extended period of time, the EMS council should periodically review the plan to assure it is representing the current EMS needs of the community or area, and is being implemented.

The planning report provides the personnel responsible for the development of the supporting communication system with the necessary operational data to identify the communication needs of the individual EMS program and their combined operation as an integrated EMS system. To provide the nontechnical personnel with a better understanding of this phase of the communication planning, Chapter 5 is provided as a review of the terms and capabilities of typical EMS communication systems.

※ *Chapter 5*

The Capabilities of EMS
Telecommunications

Before considering the EMS communication system plan itself, some of the commonly found attributes and capabilities of EMS communications will be discussed.

TERMINOLOGY

In radio communication, *simplex* refers to a system with a single channel, allowing communication between two stations in one direction only. *Duplex* is a means whereby both communication stations can simultaneously receive and transmit. *Channels* may be used to identify specific radio frequencies providing either a one-way or two-way communication. *Interface* signifies a point where transition is made between modes of operation. *Phone patch* is a means of interfacing the telephone lines with a radio system. *Terminals* are a location within a communication system where data may be injected or removed; a point of connection in an electrical circuit. (see glossary)

SYSTEM ATTRIBUTES AND CAPABILITIES

Simplex and Duplex Operation
At present, two-way radio communication is usually by simplex, meaning that only one person may talk at a time. This occurs when radio stations use only one channel. If they use two channels, one for each direction, then they are operating in duplex.

Simplex radio communications have been commonly used by public-safety agencies for reasons of economy, FCC licensing, conservation of frequencies, and simplicity of operation. The procedure of taking turns is not necessarily a detriment, but may assist in maintaining operator discipline. On a shared radio circuit, communications must be concise to be effective. By conserving channels through simplex operation, the public-safety agencies have available more separate channels of communication.

Multiplexing

To conserve the use of the limited available radio channels, it is technically possible to have more than one signal on a single channel, or group of channels. This process is known as multiplexing. There are many technical variations to these types of radio communication that are designed for specific program needs.

The telephone is the most widely available means of public communication. By a type of multiplexing, many separate transmissions can be carried simultaneously over a single telephone channel. This ability of the telephone system to handle large volumes of traffic involving both voice and data is a satisfactory means of communication, providing a wire or cable can connect the terminals of the system. When this is not practical (such as for mobile emergency vehicles or for people on the move), then radio communication is necessary. By applying interfacing techniques, the best of both communication systems can be used to the advantage of the people being served.

System Redundancy

Redundancy is required to ensure the necessary reliability of an EMS communications system. No communication system is 100 percent reliable. Equipment is complex, fragile, and exposed to environmental and usage abuse, and consequently is subject to failure. Thus, there is a need for back-up communications, which may entail direct duplication, as a radio system paralleling a telephone system, or alternative routing from one terminal to another.

Redundancy of power source, periodically tested, is also important. Communication systems are not entirely self-contained, ordinarily relying on outside resources for continuous electric power. For increased reliability, every emergency communication system station requires an emergency power source with a two-week minimum period of operation. Electrically, the system should provide an automatic changeover from commercial power to the emergency source in the event of a commercial power failure. If a generator is used, it should have an automatic exercise feature to assure operational capability when needed.

The Resource Communication Center (RCC)

The base terminal is the nerve center of a communication system. In the EMS communication center, the central emergency medical dispatcher (CMED) reacts to an emergency call, provides continuity, and follows through to the conclusion of the necessary reactions.

Of calls from the public, the immediate-action type are in the minority. It is necessary, therefore, that the communication center have emergency dispatchers trained in the proper handling of both emergency and nonemergency calls, transferring the latter to appropriate agencies.

The CMED should be trained in two fields, emergency medical care and system resource management. In the role of emergency medical care mediator, this person is responsible for determining the urgency of the call and deciding on the type of reaction required. Although, at this writing, no standards for the levels of medical training or resource management have been identified, the CMED—in order to function to the full potential of the position—must meet minimum prerequisites in both areas.

Medical training differentiates this position from those of other public-safety agencies. Other prerequisites must include an understanding of the functions of the communication equipment, the dexterity to manipulate the equipment, and the poise, self-reliance, and alertness to react in a wise and timely manner under duress.

Public Access.

The CMED may receive telephone calls concerning medical emergencies directly from citizens, or as relayed from a 911 answering service (public safety answering point—PSAP). The citizen using the 911 emergency telephone number, or the multiple-digit area number to report a medical emergency, should receive service from a CMED in not more than ten seconds.

The dispatcher has access to telephone trunk lines for incoming and outgoing calls. These may be normal subscriber lines to which every telephone has access, or they can be private or limited-access lines available only to predetermined telephone users. The center would use the latter for emergency telephone service to the terminals of the EMS system, including the base for the EMS vehicle service, the emergency department of the receiving hospital and terminals of the public-safety agencies that provide direct support. Sometimes this type of telephone service is called a hot line because it is always ready to use—no waiting. In such installations, the person removing the handset from the telephone cradle activates the bell and flashing light at the other terminal, which continue until the call is answered.

Telephone calls coming into the EMS communication center over a 911 line may have the *hold and re-ring* feature. The hold feature prevents the caller from making a disconnect by hanging up the telephone handset before the dispatcher has all of the necessary data from the caller. If the caller does hang up, the dispatcher can *re-ring* the caller's telephone. Only the dispatcher can disconnect the calling telephone from the 911 telephone line. This feature also enables the dispatcher to call back on suspected false reports or to verify data, especially location.

In times of a community disaster, there could be an overload of the 911 telephone system. To prevent a citizen from unnecessarily tying up the 911 telephone circuits, the dispatcher can make a forced disconnect and free the telephone lines for more urgent calls.

Another time-saver that the telephone company can make available in conjunction with the 911 emergency telephone service is the dial-tone-first service that can be extended to coin-operated telephones. This feature enables a citizen to dial the 911 emergency telephone number from a public telephone booth without first depositing a coin. This service, like the 911 emergency telephone service, has not been made available nationwide, at this writing.

Basically, the radio communication equipment in the EMS communication center provides two-way voice and data communications with mobile radio units and fixed radio terminals in the EMS communication system. Radio equipment is also used as back-up communications for critical telephone lines in the event of a failure or overload in times of a large disaster. Terminal-to-terminal communications from the EMS communication center to the public-safety agencies may be by telephone, radio, or both, depending on the local situation—distances involved, reliability of the telephone system, allowable procedures for interagency communications, and so on.

The police departments in many cities use electronic devices for record-keeping. Similarly, EMS data may be maintained in a computer and accessed by the dispatcher on a video screen. Data applicable to the duties of the CMED should include the status of EMS vehicles, display of community and area maps, telephone numbers, radio frequencies, availability of hospital facilities, and the like (see Figure 5-1).

Tape recorders are used to record the dispatcher's and caller's conversations over the telephone and radio systems in the communication center. These recordings are very important as administrative and legal records.

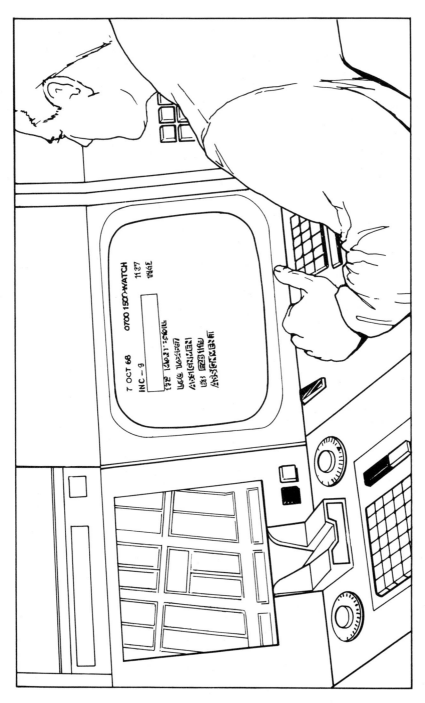

Figure 5-1. Typical Dispatcher's Console Display.

When an emergency call indicates the need for an emergency medical vehicle, the CMED must ascertain the type of emergency involved—cardiac, burns, auto accident, fall, drowning, and so on. Where there is a selection of emergency medical vehicle services within the community, the CMED must know the life-saving and emergency medical capability of the EMTs and their equipment.

Once the EMTs are alerted to a medical emergency, they first need the *location* of the emergency. The vehicle should be rolling in not more than 30 seconds. By using radio communication between the CMED at the communication center and the vehicle as it is en route to the scene of the emergency, the CMED can provide the attendants with additional information on the location, road conditions, special approaches, the medical complaint, and any updated additional available data.

The system's early response may or may not anticipate a hospital delivery. Once it is confirmed that a receiving emergency department (ED) hospital delivery is to be made, the patient, medical consultant, EMT or CMED should select the receiving hospital and advise them of this fact. In areas where there are emergency department choices, considerations include the EMTs' or physician's diagnosis and prognosis, degree of patient stabilization, distances to be traveled, and the patient's physician's request. Obviously this requires some degree of *receiving hospital* categorization.

When the selected emergency department has been alerted, a radio channel may be identified and used for hospital vehicle communication. The CMED continues to monitor the channel to be aware of any changing condition in the patient that would affect the delivery plan, or any delay in the delivery—such as an accident—that would require additional support.

In some rural areas there may not be a choice of medical facilities to accept the patient; at best these may have minimal capabilities. If such limited facilities are used to stabilize a patient for transport to a distant hospital, then the system must include that hospital. This can tax the ingenuity of the CMED and the other personnel involved. Pre-planning at all levels (including physicians) can provide a degree of assurance that the decisions made under duress will provide the optimal use of available medical resources.

Rural Operations

The early alerting of the CMED to an incident is important anywhere, but especially in the rural area. Here, there is a higher death rate per accident than in urban areas, and two of the contributing factors appear to be delay in discovery of the incident and lack of means of alerting the emergency medical system.

In rural areas, pre-hospital care and stabilization are even more critical because of the greater distances to the scene, as well as to the receiving hospital emergency department. The emergency vehicle's medical care equipment, the training of the EMTs, and the mobile and portable radio voice communication with the hospital emergency department physician are all critical services that are especially important in providing the necessary pre-hospital patient care in the rural environment. Where there is a long transport time from the scene of the incident to the hospital emergency department, there is an even *greater* requirement for the constant monitoring of the patient's vital signs, and the capability to maintain a satisfactory level of stabilization.

Radio Communications

In the radio frequency spectrum, the Federal Communications Commission (FCC) has designated certain VHF and UHF radio frequencies for the use of emergency medical services. In a given area, some of these frequencies are shared. Thus, when a medical emergency mission is begun, the emergency vehicle and the hospital are assigned communication channels to be used at the time, and establish their priority for the duration of the run.* Frequencies in the VHF band and some in the UHF band provide simplex and repeater operation, while selected frequencies in the UHF band permit duplex operation (see Chapter 8). This use of two radio frequencies enables the two terminals to select from several modes of communication, such as using duplex voice, or using one channel for simplex voice and one for telemetry. Depending on the kinds of terminal equipment in use, many different types of communications can be used to best satisfy the needs of the emergency situation.

Radio communications between the scene of the emergency and other support elements can involve several terminals, and be quite sophisticated. An additional radio communication may be with an air-mobile intensive-care unit (helicopter or fixed-wing aircraft) to expedite the transport of a critical patient to the receiving hospital. There may be the need for a second (back-up) supporting EMS vehicle. Depending on the availability of radio channels in the area, the additional EMS support terminals may share the frequencies established for their mission, or use additional frequencies. In medical emergencies involving several elements, radio communication enables the consulting physician to direct and supervise the treatment and medication of the patient by EMTs at the scene and during

---

*Appendix A, entitled The Federal Communications Commission and EMS, provides greater detail on the operation of the Commission in the allocation of radio frequencies.

transport to the hospital, either from the hospital emergency department or elsewhere, using a portable or mobile two-way radio.

In addition, there may be the need for support from other public-safety agencies. Police officers may be needed for traffic control, firemen may be required to extricate victims or prevent a fire. Rescue units that provide special recovery and support services may be called. Tow trucks may be needed to move a damaged vehicle. All of these support services use communications to be alerted and, once they are involved, to provide coordination of their activities with other agencies.

The CMED at the EMS communication center is a key person in all of this activity. The communication resource, functions effectively when there is central control to coordinate efforts. The consulting physician provides the medical direction for the care of the patient. The CMED provides the control of the communication system, which provides for coordination of the many elements. Without this means of timely coordination, the full life-saving potential of the EMS system could not be realized.

EMS COORDINATION

Coordination within the EMS System

The emergency medical communications network ties together the various functions of the total EMS system. Since all agencies participating in the EMS system are interdependent, interagency cooperation and coordination is necessary for an effective communications network. This coordination through communications is graphically illustrated in Figure 5-2.

The Organizational Position of EMS in Public Safety

For years the public has called the police or fire departments for any emergency service. These were the community's public-safety agencies; ambulance companies and hospitals were not so considered. As a result, emergency medical service was usually requested only after fire or police personnel had arrived at the scene of the emergency, evaluated the situation, and had reported to their headquarters the need for an ambulance. Where this pattern has continued to prevail, perhaps involving administration of first aid by fire or police personnel, the life-saving potential of emergency medical services are drastically reduced.

Today, however, EMS is recognized—together with police and fire—as an essential public-safety service. Organizationally, as Figure 5-2 illustrates, an EMS system is not self-contained, as are police

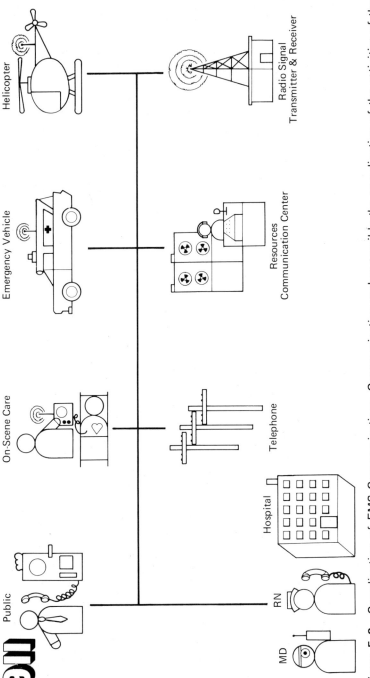

Figure 5–2. Coordination of EMS Communications. Communication makes possible the coordination of the activities of the emergency medical service system. The communication center provides the interface of radio and telephone communications between the elements of the system. The dispatcher receives incoming emergency medical calls, dispatches emergency vehicles, and alerts other elements of the system.

and fire departments, but is broadly inclusive, encompassing a wide spectrum of related services and disciplines. The need for close coordination and cooperation, not only among agencies within the EMS system but also among all public-safety agencies, is being increasingly recognized as essential if the citizen's welfare is to be adequately served. Communication systems linking these agencies, the development of 911, the PSAP, and consolidated dispatch centers are both the result of this recognition and a means for furthering cooperation. This is illustrated in Figure 5-3.

The Position of the CMED

The position of the dispatcher for the EMS communication system (that is, the CMED), and the dispatchers for the other public-safety agencies in the community, are shown in Figure 5-4. When the dispatchers for the three agencies are co-tenants of a single communication center, the response time for service can be minimized.

The CMED occupies a key position in the EMS system, and receives all emergency medical calls from the public or other public agencies, and is responsible for making a judgmental and timely decision on the needed response. Errors in judgment or delays in reacting could have fatal consequences. During times of crisis or disaster, when dispatchers are under great pressure, it is particularly important to have sufficient and appropriate communications. There must be an adequate number of dispatcher operating positions designed into the RCC. It must also have enough terminals, with the necessary priorities, to coordinate agencies and system components to avoid delays. This is illustrated in Figure 5-5.

Rural Communities

In many rural communities with limited populations, the public-safety agencies cannot economically justify the personnel, equipment, and facilities identified in the preceding illustrations. These communities, however, may be part of a larger catchment area and depend on the adjoining public-safety agencies within the area for additional support. For instance, the rural dispatcher may work during daylight hours, and turn nighttime dispatching to a nearby urban CMED. An emergency public-safety communication center of this type is illustrated in Figure 5-6. Here, a single-position dispatcher has telephone and radio access to all of the public-safety agencies, either within the community or in the larger catchment area.

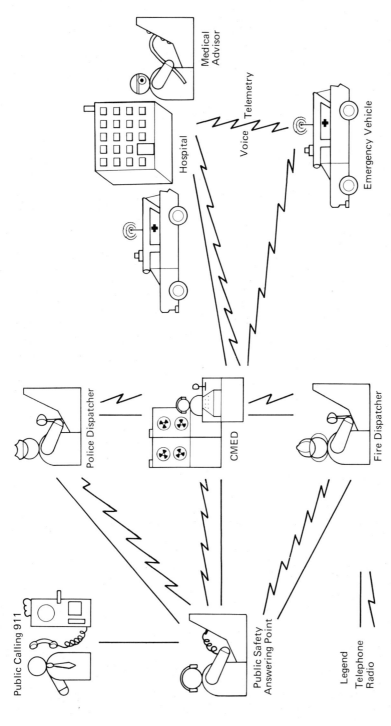

Figure 5-3. Emergency Medical Service Communication System. Responding to a citizens telephone call for emergency medical care.

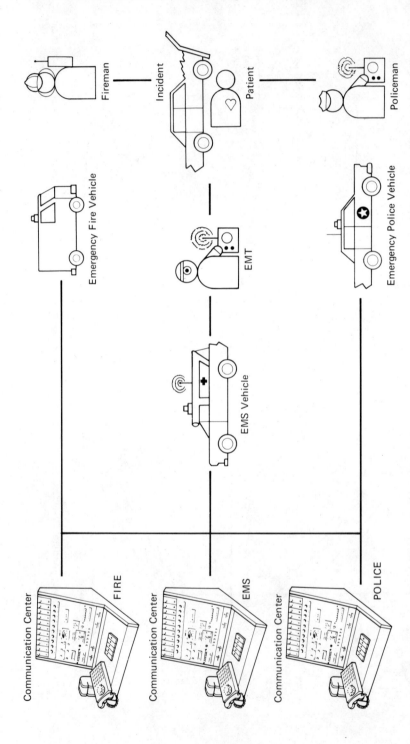

Figure 5-4. Contenent Operation Public Safety Services. Contenant Operation of the EMS Communication Center, Police and Fire Departments Communications Centers Provides the Community with an Emergency Service Resource Communication Center.

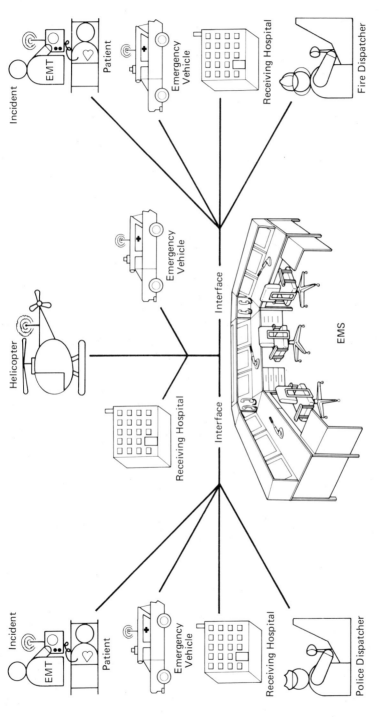

Figure 5-5. Multiple Position RCC. A multiple position emergency service resource communications center for maximum of three central medical emergency dispatchers operating simultaneously from control panels having multiple appearances of incoming and outgoing calls.

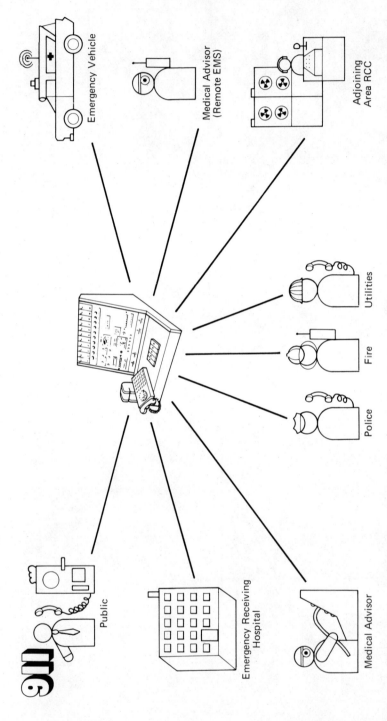

Figure 5–6. Emergency Service Resource Communication Center. A one operator position RCC for responding to all incoming requests for emergency service by the use of radio and telephone communications to emergency vehicle service, emergency receiving hospital, medical advisor (at hospital or remote), fire, police and utility departments, and to adjoining emergency service RCC's.

A Case Study

The following purely hypothetical case study is offered as an example of a typical series of communications that accomplish entry into the system. These make possible appropriate handling, including emergency medical treatment—at the scene and intransit—and final disposition. It is offered as a "walk-through" of the system, which allows one to see the sequential steps by which a person requests and receives emergency pre-hospital treatment.

Time	Communicator	Message or Action
8:10	Citizen:	Get me an ambulance (collapses).
	Bystander:	Who do you want me to call?
	Citizen:	Anyone. Just get help (becomes unconscious).
8:11	Bystander:	(Goes into nearby drugstore; dials 911 [or whatever the local number is for medical emergencies]. The 911 operator answers after one ring, and pushes a button connecting the caller with the EMS operator.)
8:11	911 Operator:	Emergency Services. Do you need police, fire, or medical help?
	Bystander:	Medical help.
	EMS operator:	Give me your location and phone number. (The phone number is necessary in case the EMS operator has to call back for more information.)
8:12	Bystander:	I'm on Green Street, near 7th Avenue. This is 377-7777
8:12	EMS operator:	You're on Green Street near 7th Avenue. (Operator repeats location to verify correctness.) Is it north or south of 7th Avenue?
	Bystander:	Just a little south of 7th Avenue, near the drug store.
8:13	EMS operator:	(Hands dispatch card to dispatcher.)* Is the victim conscious? About how old?

*In this example, in which the use of 911 is assumed, the apparent additional seconds added to the process by the interposition of two operators between the caller and the dispatcher is more than compensated for by the time saved by having a single, toll-free number clearly posted on the pay phone.

Time	Communicator	Message or Action
	Bystander:	He seems to be unconscious; a man, black, about 60. (EMS operator passes additional information to the dispatcher.)
8:14	EMS operator:	We have dispatched a mobile intensive care vehicle. It should be there in about 4 minutes from now.
8:13	Dispatcher:	Rescue 3—Man down—Green near 7th Avenue—exact location slightly south of 7th Avenue on Green near drug store—victim is male, approximately 50-60 years old–no further information.
	Rescue 3:	Affirmative. Green, slightly south of 7th Avenue near drug store. Am proceeding.
8:14	Dispatcher:	Rescue 3—Further information indicates victim has been in this condition for several minutes and is not moving at this time. Standing by.
	Rescue 3:	Affirmative. (There is now, ideally, a run time of less than 5 minutes.)
8:18	Rescue 3:	Am on the scene. There is a crowd. Request police assistance. Over.
	Dispatcher:	Affirmative. Police being dispatched.
	Rescue 3:	Affirmative.
8:20	Rescue 3:	Blank Hospital, this is Rescue 3 on Med 1. Over.*
	Hospital:	Blank Hospital. Go ahead Rescue 3.
	Rescue 3:	We have an approximately 60-year-old male who collapsed; we have no further medical history. Vital signs are B-P 180 over 100, pulse rate 120 and irregular, respirations 24 and shallow, victim is black. Conjunctiva and buccal mucosa appear somewhat cyanotic, although it is difficult to tell. Stand by for electrocardiogram.

---

*Each UHF Med channel has two frequencies, one on which the rescue unit transmits and the hospital receives, and one on which the hospital transmits and the rescue unit receives.

Time	Communicator	Message or Action
	Hospital:	Affirmative. Standing by.
	Rescue 3:	(There then follows approximately 30 seconds of electrocardiographic rhythm strip.) Do you receive? Over
	Hospital:	Rescue 3, this is Dr. Smith at Blank Hospital. We have a clear tracing which shows atrial fibrillation with numerous premature ventricular contractions. Suggest you start an I-V with dextrose 5 percent in water immediately. Let us know as soon as the I-V has been started and at that time give us a repeat rhythm strip.*
8:22	Rescue 3:	Affirmative.
	Rescue 3:	Blank Hospital, stand by for repeat rhythm strip and repeat vital signs.
	Hospital:	Standing by.
	Rescue 3:	(There then follows a 30-second rhythm strip which shows continued atrial fibrillation with even more frequent premature ventricular contractions.) On repeat vital signs, we show a B-P of 200 over 100. Pulse rate continues to be 120 and irregular. Breathing 22 and shallow. I-V is running. Over.
	Dr. Smith:	Is your victim still unconscious? Over.
	Rescue 3:	The victim is beginning to rouse and is groaning, and pointing to his chest. Over.
8:24	Dr. Smith:	Can you hear breath sounds, and describe to me? Over.
	Rescue 3;	They are quite distant and would appear to be fine, crackling rales over most of the lung field, especially on inspiration. Over.

---

*In most systems, invasive treatments, such as intravenous administrations, can be given by paramedics only when specifically authorized by a physician.

Time	*Communicator*	*Message or Action*
	Dr. Smith:	Give morphine—repeat, morphine, 1 milligram at a time at about 30-second intervals, checking B-P after each milligram up to approximately 5 milligrams. Pressure should go down, and breathing improve. Have patient in semi-sitting position with oxygen. Over.
8:29	Rescue 3:	(Repeats instructions verbatim.) Proceeding as instructed. Should we use rotating tourniquets? Over.
	Dr. Smith:	Affirmative on tourniquets. (Pause period.)
8:30	Rescue 3:	Rescue 3 calling Blank Hospital.
	Hospital:	Dr. Smith, go ahead.
	Rescue 3:	The pressure has come down to 160 over 90. Color appears to be better and patient is now conscious. Have name, address, and further details; victim states that he is a visitor and knows no one in the city. Has had a known heart condition in the past and takes nitroglycerin occasionally. Over.
	Dr. Smith:	Affirmative. Would like another rhythm strip. Over.
	Rescue 3:	Affirmative. (Another rhythm strip which shows atrial fibrillation, but with only an occasional premature ventricular contraction.) Do you receive? Over.
8:31	Dr. Smith:	Affirmative. Begin transport with patient in semi-sitting position receiving oxygen and being monitored. If pulse rate gets more irregular, pressure changes, or other change in symptoms, advise. Over.
	Rescue 3:	Affirmative. Beginning transport 8:32. Will proceed to Blank Hospital. Estimated time of arrival 8:41. Over.

Time	Communicator	Message or Action
	Dr. Smith:	Affirmative. Standing by for arrival.
8:32	Rescue 3:	Beginning transport.
8:38	Rescue 3:	Rescue 3 calling Blank Hospital.
	Hospital:	Blank Hospital. Go ahead.
	Rescue 3:	We are about 3 minutes from the hospital. Can report a pressure of 140 over 90, but with considerable irregularity of the pulse. Am sending a repeat EKG. (20-second strip reveals multifocal premature ventricular contractions with runs of ventricular tachycardia.) Over.
	Dr. Smith	Give 50 milligrams, that's five zero milligrams, lidocaine, slowly. Over.
8:39	Rescue 3:	(Repeating instructions verbatim.) Affirmative.
8:40	Rescue 3:	(One minute later.) We are about 1 minute from the hospital and am sending a repeat rhythm strip. Over. (Rhythm strip shows abolition of premature ventricular contractions and ventricular tachycardia.)
	Dr. Smith:	Your EKG shows good effect of the lidocaine. Any other changes in patient condition? Over.
	Rescue 3:	Negative. Over.
	Dr. Smith:	Proceed. Over.
8:42	Rescue 3:	This is Rescue 3 arriving at Blank Hospital. Over.
	Dispatcher:	Affirmative.
8:58	Rescue 3:	This is Rescue 3 reporting ready for service, 8:58.

(Rescue 3 has assisted in the first few minutes of overlapping care at Blank Hospital Emergency Department. They have transmitted all of the vital information to Dr. Smith. They have turned in a copy of their run report to the hospital so that all treatment and effect is now known by the emergency department physician and nurses at Blank Hospital. They have stood by as part of their learning experience for several minutes to observe the early treatment of the victim. The victim is now doing well and headed for coronary care, where he is expected to recover. They have prepared their vehicle and equipment for the next call.

This is a typical transaction showing the access, on-line medical treatment, and final disposition of a case at the receiving hospital. Total elapsed time was 47 minutes. We hope that by presenting such a case study some of the special considerations for emergency medical communication have become more apparent. Some cases are simpler than this; many are much more complicated.

Calls from the public for emergency medical service are predominantly by telephone using an emergency number such as 911 or a seven-digit emergency number. Some calls are received by radio communications initiated by an observer of a medical emergency, as a police patrolman, taxi driver, truck driver, or the public using CB or other amateur radio equipment. Whatever the means of communication, they are received by the public-safety answering point (PSAP) operator who receives all public requests for emergency assistance, regardless of type. The PSAP operator's immediate response to the caller is "Medical, fire, or police?" If medical, the call is connected to the operator of the emergency medical service communication center who talks to the caller long enough to determine the needed response. If it requires ambulance service, the dispatcher touches a switch that connects to an emergency telephone and public-address system in the alert room of the rescue squad, where EMTs are waiting for a call. Upon receiving the location of the medical emergency, the EMTs and vehicle leave on their call. Additional details on the emergency are transmitted by the dispatcher to the EMTs as they are en route to the scene of the emergency.

If the caller provides sufficient details of the medical emergency, the dispatcher will notify the hospital emergency room that will be receiving the patient and advise the EMTs where to take the patient. If the details are obtained at the scene by the EMTs, this information is transmitted to the dispatcher who in turn, advises the emergency department (ED) concerned. If appropriate, the dispatcher will advise the ED of the radio frequency to use when communicating with the EMTs on the call.

At the scene, the EMTs assess the emergency and, within their capability, perform the necessary treatment and medical services to sufficiently stabilize the patient preparatory to transport to the appropriate receiving facility. If the medical emergency requires support from other public-safety agencies, such as the police and fire departments, the dispatcher immediately communicates with these departments. Voice radio communication is established between the EMTs and the receiving medical staff to apprise them of the patient's condition, the extent of the medical emergency services rendered, and expected time at transport and of arrival at the hospital.

If the patient's condition is critical during transport, the dialog between the receiving physician at the hospital and the EMTs concerning treatment and medication will continue by radio communication, as in our example.

The receiving physician in a hospital emergency department also needs communication *within* the hospital to request assistance, obtain supplies, and consult with his peers or the administrative staff.

The records of the vital signs observed, and the treatment and medication administered to the patient by the EMTs, are given to the receiving physician. This normally completes the responsibilities of the EMTs for a run. They advise the dispatcher of the time they completed the run and of their availability. If no other run is required, the EMS vehicle is returned to the duty station and the EMTs return to the alert room.

The preceding illustration of the operation of the emergency medical service communication system involved a public call for emergency medical care. While the dialogue of the preceding case study may be typical, it is secondary to the objective, that is, the sequential steps taken by the personnel in the EMS system when responding to a public request for medical service. There is no prescribed dialogue for communication between the parties When the communication system is a simplex design, it is practical for the person speaking to conclude with some type of indicator, thus allowing the other person to talk. The word 'over' is commonly used. Obviously, on full duplex systems this is not a prerequisite. In like manner, acknowledgment of a request for service may take several forms; affirmative is used in the preceding case study. However, the words "I copy," "confirm," or many others could be used. The objective in word selection is to use one that is not readily confused with a similarly pronounced word. Not all radio communication has the clarity and noise-free operation of the telephone service. To avoid misunderstanding when communicating under adverse conditions, word selection and repetition are important to the success of the communication. Many of the words selected were developed in the military radio service and among radio amateur operators, and have carried over to other radio services.

The preceding illustration of the operation of the emergency medical service communication system involved a public call for emergency medical care. The call was handled entirely within the EMS system. However, a major source of calls for emergency medical service will be from the police and fire departments to the EMS communication center. Coordination of EMS support activities from these departments can be effected with a minimal loss of time, and response time can be minimized when the dispatchers for these three community emergency services are cotenants of a single communication center.

This chapter has provided a nontechnical insight to some of the terminology associated with radio communication systems, followed by the types of support a communication system can provide to EMS programs. The next chapter continues the subject by identifying specific communication requirements needed in the development of a communications plan.

Chapter 6

The Communications Plan

Although the number and types of communication hardware items used in a given system, as well as their configuration, will depend on local circumstances, it may be useful to review the various common functions any EMS communication system must serve. Such considerations must be addressed in the process of establishing an effective EMS plan.

ACCESS

The system must provide an easy method for anyone to call for emergency medical help. Ordinarily this is by telephone; on major highways this may be supplemented by roadside call boxes; in remote areas by CB radio, radios supplied to highway users, or other means.

In most localities notification of an emergency is likely to be delayed: (1) because the caller is faced with a multiplicity of emergency numbers—hospitals, fire and police departments, rescue squads, private ambulance companies; and (2) because the caller does not have the proper coin for a pay phone. If the time gap between the event and the notification is large, the patient may die, no matter how fast the response time of the system.

A primary requirement of an EMS system is, therefore, that there be a single, clearly posted number, readily available to any telephone user, for emergency medical help in a given area. Ideally this number should be toll-free. At present, EMS systems employ, variously, 911, a single 7-digit number, a Wats or 800 number, dial Zero, a single police or fire department number, or separate consolidated dispatch or emergency medical numbers in different sectors of an EMS system.

Adoption of 911 as a national all-emergency toll-free number has become national policy by publication of the Office of Telecommunication Policy (OTP) Bulletin No. 73-1 (Selected Reference No. 15). Local adoption has been rather spotty. Florida and California have mandated its use by 1978 and 1982, respectively. As of January 1, 1976, 609 localities, mostly single cities or counties, were using 911 or were scheduled for this service in the near future. The discrepancy between national and local policy has been variously attributed to a reluctance of emergency response organizations (fire, police, volunteer squads, commercial ambulance companies) to cooperate; to the inability of small, often multiple, local telephone companies to provide the service; or to the high cost estimate supplied by the telephone company for the conversion. On the other hand, in many of those areas that do not now have 911, this number will reach an operator who can connect the caller to an emergency service.

Telephone calls to 911 are intended to provide the public with direct access to an emergency switchboard operated and staffed by local government public safety agencies organized to respond to all types of emergencies on a community-wide basis. The telephone company provides the 911 service to a single public safety answering point (PSAP) in the community that will answer all 911 calls and immediately transfer them to the appropriate dispatcher—fire, police, or EMS.

The advantages of this system are obvious. As spelled out in Office of Telecommunication Policy (OTP) Bulletin [15]:

A clear need that all citizens be able rapidly to summon help in an emergency situation has long been recognized. A communications system which is immediately available and easy to use can help to meet this need. A person should be able to call for police, fire, rescue, and other emergency aid promptly and without confusion, and without regard to his familiarity with a particular community.

Some providers of emergency aid are concerned about an increase in notification time resulting from the interposition of the PSAP in the access chain. This objection ignores the greater overall saving of time from having a single universally available number. The *OTP Bulletin* [15] states that "a secondary objective should be to enable public safety agencies to satisfy their operational and communications needs more efficiently." That this is actually the case can be borne out by the experiences of localities such as Hermiston, Oregon; Victoria, Texas; and Philadelphia, which have 911 and consolidated dispatch. But considerable discussion and debate in the EMS council stressing the time saved from event to notification by using 911 may be needed to carry this point.

EMS systems that as yet have been unable to use 911 have adopted a variety of substitutes. Most commonly they use a single 7-digit number going only to the CMED. Tie-lines from the RCC to the police and fire dispatchers ensure rapid transfer to the CMED of emergency medical calls coming to those agencies. Some systems use an 800- or in-WATS number; others instruct emergency callers to dial the operator. In rural areas the sheriff's office, retaining its number, often becomes the consolidated dispatch point for the county. The nature of such an alternative access number is less important than the ease and efficiency with which it can be used. In any event, such an alternative should be used only as an interim measure pending establishment of 911.

Another effort has been the organization of the users of Channel 9 (27.065 MHz) of the Citizens Band, designated by the FCC for motorist assistance and emergency use only. One CB club, with the encouragement and support of the state health department and the governor, has organized a network of CB base stations for reporting medical emergencies. Residents and visitors with CB radios are provided with maps indicating base station locations, and with a list of the stations, indicating monitoring hours and frequencies. At this writing about 400 base stations are in operation in that state. Base station volunteers are provided with a standard list of questions to ensure a measure of quality control. When a base station operator has verified an emergency, the information is relayed by a toll-free 800-number to the state Crisis Center, which can then dispatch the nearest available ambulance or appropriate emergency vehicle using the statewide microwave EMS network.

In another state, during the first six months of a program whereby the state highway patrol has been monitoring CB, over 6,000 reports of traffic accidents were received, with an average notification time of 9 minutes, versus an approximately 15-minute average for reporting by telephone. In addition, the highway patrol received approximately 50,000 other CB notifications regarding traffic and criminal violations, dangerous road conditions, and requests for assistance.

The usefulness of Channel 9 for emergency medical communications is limited, however, by the extremely large class of licensees among whom its use must be shared, technical problems such as skip interference, the limited transmitter power permitted (5 watts), and the lack of protection from interference by licensees who mis-use the channel. Proper use of the channel is difficult to enforce, and licensees are not tested for their competence.

RESPONSE

A resource communications center (RCC) where a dispatcher—a CMED trained in emergency care and in communications—controls the ambulance flow and EMS communications within a defined area is the essential key to prompt response. Ideally this is one central dispatch office for an EMS region. Some EMS systems, such as those based in Kansas City, Missouri and Lafayette, Louisiana have shown that this can be done even in large, multicounty regions. Some multicounty rural systems have adopted the expedient of several subordinate dispatch points, usually one per county located in the county sheriff's office. In sparsely settled rural areas the medical number may ring directly in the homes of EMTs, or the initial response may be by specially trained quick-response units of local citizens.

The mode by which the CMED notifies an ambulance crew of a medical emergency will depend on local circumstances. Most commonly this is by direct landline to the ambulance station, often with the dispatcher's voice coming over a loudspeaker. If an ambulance is returning to base from a run, or if ambulances are dispersed about an area for quick response, the dispatching may be directly by radio to the rescue squad. In areas where volunteers provides rescue service, the dispatcher may activate pagers carried by squad members to as-semble the squad.

Basic CMED communications, then, include those transmitted on dedicated telephone lines to ambulance stations and hospitals, direct radio communication with ambulances, and tie lines to other emergency services. Redundancy is important to allow for equipment failure: whenever possible, landlines should be paralleled by radio links. Links to Civil Defense and to adjacent EMS systems for disaster coordination are also important. Finally, CMED equipment should include a means of recording all system radio and telephone traffic, both for monitoring for system improvement and for legal protection.

Other communication devices that can aid the CMED include automatic location identification (ALI) and automatic number identification (ANI) for pinpointing calls; a display board, manual or automatic, showing ambulance locations; computerized data retrieval of information on hospital or rescue squad capabilities (or, in a few systems, on patient histories); telephone hold or ring-back, enabling the dispatcher to keep in touch or reestablish contact with the caller; or computerized display of dispatch information for sub-regional dispatch centers.

Again, the complexity and configuration of the communications design (and the training of the dispatcher) will vary with local circumstances and with the role assigned to the CMED. A system with a single ambulance company providing only basic emergency care will need less complicated communications than one in which, for instance, mobile intensive-care units (MICUs) respond to critical cases, volunteer EMT-Basic squads to other medical emergencies, and commercial ambulances to transport calls. In a system where dispatching is done at subregional dispatch centers, the role of the central communications office may be one only of monitoring and support coordination. At the other extreme are systems in which all communication, including telemetry, is routed through the CMED, who also governs channel allocation among system components on a real-time basis and arranges doctor talk.

The most important consideration for EMS planners is that they provide, in the communications section of the EMS plan, an accurate definition of what the communications system must do if it is to serve the medical needs of the area.

AMBULANCE-HOSPITAL COMMUNICATIONS

A basic requirement in an EMS system is that ambulance crews be able to communicate with hospital personnel, to alert the emergency department (ED) at the hospital of an impending arrival and to get medical advice on treatment at the scene and in transit. Basic options relate to the structure of the communications design and to the degree of communications sophistication desired.

The design structure may entail either direct radio transmissions between the ambulance and the hospital base station, or transmissions between the ambulance and CMED, with the traffic patched by landline from CMED to the hospital. The former gives the hospital somewhat more flexibility in communications at the relatively minor cost of a base station, and requires ED doctors and nurses to become familiar with radio operation. The latter provides stronger central control of communications, and provides nothing more complicated than a telephone handset for use by ED personnel.

The question of equipment sophistication is likely to revolve around the desirability of telemetry. At this writing, the subject is being widely debated. Many physicians regard telemetry as essential for management of cardiac cases, particularly in areas where ambulance runs can be long; some feel that telemetry should be used in every life-threatening incident. On the other hand, in areas where local physicians have trained paramedics and subsequently worked closely with them and know their capabilities, it is often felt that voice communication between physician and paramedic renders telemetry unnecessary. While telemetry requires employment of paramedics, the reverse it not true: paramedics can read the vital signs and ECG, advising the physician by voice radio of the result.

Because the FCC has allocated just eight UHF-frequency Med channels, urban EMS planners will have to use particular care in designing their system configuration and operational procedures to avoid channel congestion and interference. In such circumstances, core coordination and RCC channel control assume special importance.

As with telemetry itself, medical opinion is divided on the issue of continuous versus intermittant transmission of telemetry data. The former provides an unbroken indication and record of the patient's condition, but ties up one channel during the run and requires use of another channel for voice transmissions; the latter permits voice transmissions alternately with telemetry and permits the physician to monitor, if necessary, more than one telemetry transmission. Multiplexing of telemetry and voice communications affords more effective use of a single channel.

Another option commonly used is the hand-held transceiver, which permits EMTs to maintain radio communications, directly or via a vehicular repeater in the ambulance, while they are away from the ambulance. Conversely, physicians with such sets can advise the EMTs and monitor some vital signs from any location within range.

INTRA-HOSPITAL COMMUNICATIONS

The functions that must be served by communications within a hospital include: (1) doctor paging; (2) communication between the emergency department and the various critical-care units; and (3) priority handling of emergency cases.

Doctor paging is particularly important in hospitals that do not have 24-hour physician coverage of the emergency department. Within the hospital, this may be accomplished by intercom, a public-address system, or low-frequency or VHF pagers. For physicians outside the hospital, radio pagers or hand-held transceivers can be used. The latter have the dual advantages of being able to provide the doctor immediately with the necessary information about the emergency, and of enabling that person to talk directly with the rescue squad, from whatever their location.

Communications between the emergency department and critical-care units, burn units, or other special emergency-care services can be by hotline telephone or intercom; in either case, these communication facilities should not be available for other uses.

Priority handling of emergency calls that come directly to the hospital may require modification of the hospital switchboard to enable the hospital operator, if it is necessary, to patch such a call directly to the CMED.

INTER-HOSPITAL COMMUNICATIONS

Interhospital communications, primarily for patient transfer and disaster coordination, can be by commercial telephone, radio, or by hotlines patched at the radio control center, depending on the urgency of the call. Many hospitals have long been members of local interhospital radio networks. The CMED should have the ability to monitor such networks, and, in time of disaster, to control the traffic.

This chapter provided data on the application of specific types of communication facilities to EMS program requirements, and established the basis for developing a communications plan. The next sequence in the planning process is the technical design of a basic EMS communication system. The next chapter, however, temporarily deviates from the sequence to introduce the communications consultant. This can be timely to acquaint the EMS council with the services that can be provided by the consultant, techniques of personnel selection, contracting, evaluating, and related subjects.

Chapter 7

Consultants

WHO THE CONSULTANTS ARE

An electronic communication consultant—an expert in electronic communication systems engineering—is qualified to provide professional counsel on a fee basis. Most states have established qualifying requirements for registering engineering consultants as professional engineers (PE), and issue licenses to operate in the state. Legitimate consultants have no commercial affiliation with manufacturers, equipment suppliers, or contractors. They sell only their knowledge, judgment, service, and time. EMS electronic communication consultants apply their expertise and professional experience to the field of emergency medical service. Their advice should enable the EMS committee to achieve a higher degree of excellence in a minimum of time and with a high degree of cost effectiveness.

State examining boards may provide a list of licensed professional engineers, and can assist in identifying a person or organization that meets the requirements of the EMS committee. Local, state, and federal engineering societies may assist in providing a list of prospective consultants. Other EMS organizations can usually recommend consultants that have successfully counseled them. Ask prospective consultants for a list of all of their clients and contact them for recommendations.

THE INTERVIEW

The EMS committee should prepare a standard presentation for all prospective consultants. The meeting may start with a presentation of the EMS plans and objectives, using maps, charts, and texts as applicable. Allow time for questioning by members. Present organizational charts of participating agencies, identifying key personnel with whom the consultant may have contact. Identify known and anticipated problem areas. Provide a description of communications being used by the present EMS system. Identify the known deficiencies in the system and desired kinds of communication, in technical terms. Provide sufficient detail, including diverse opinions among committee members, constraints, methods of project funding, and related data. Site visits should be arranged.

A competent consultant will not suggest solutions until all of the parameters of the problems are identified and the requirements and objectives are agreed upon. Be wary of the consultant who agrees with all of the given statements without constructive comment, and promises to solve all of your problems. The consultant should demonstrate an understanding of the problem areas. This may result in the consultant spending additional time with the committee members to get more detailed information.

PROPOSALS

As a result of the interviews, the committee selects two or three of the consultants and asks them to submit written proposals. The proposals should include the following:

1. *A redefinition of the problem or problems.* It is most important that everyone is communicating on this point.
2. *A restatement of the committee objectives.* They should be precise and include any special requirements for or constraints on the project.
3. *A proposed program.* This should identify the step-by-step approach to be used to meet committee objectives.
4. *Provisions for a review of the project.* This review is done by the committee at the completion of each phase to ensure the objectives are being met.
5. *A time schedule of the project.*
6. *The estimated cost of the project.* This would include any special consideration such as periods of payment.
7. *The benefits of the project.* These are identified in terms of increased operating efficiency, cost savings, and personnel benefits.

This list of minimum items to be included in each proposal provides a basis for comparative analysis by the committee. It is important that the consultants' proposals be treated as confidential, and those not accepted returned to the originator.

CONTRACT

When the committee has selected the consultant, a meeting should be held between the parties involved to agree on the contractual arrangements. The committee should have an input to these arrangements to assure control of the project at all times. As an example, the project may have several sequential phases with checkpoints as it is developed. The first phase may be the concept design. Succeeding phases may be the detailed design, including *operational analysis* (the means by which the requirements of the concept design are to be accomplished); *failure analysis* (a study of the required major equipment to determine a balance between the anticipated life span of the communication system and the economical life span of the equipment); *maintenance analysis* (to determine the kind and extent of maintenance required as related to the previous analyses); and a *cost analysis* that brings it all together (a cost identity of each of the desired system concepts, the operational equipment and personnel related thereto, and the recurring costs to maintain the system in consonance with the concept design).

The contractual arrangements should be for only one phase at a time, with an optional renewal clause permitting the committee to accept each phase of the project before authorizing the contract to extend to the next phase. This enables the committee to retain control of the project, and change consultants if necessary, to obtain the most qualified person or consulting firm on each phase of the project. Qualified consultants, or consulting firms, have no qualms about agreeing to this type of contract.

PROJECT DIRECTOR

A committee project director should be assigned as coordinator between the committee and the consultant. The selection of the committee project director is crucial. This director must be in accord with the selection of the consultant, be authorized to make decisions that are in accord with the contract, have ready access to needed information, and assist in expediting actions. Consideration should be given to providing the consultant with selected in-house services instead of paying the consultant for such necessities as office space, secretarial assistance, reproduction, and related services.

The committee project director must closely monitor the work of the consultant, and confer on progress, delays, contract deviation, disagreements, or related items. Unresolved items should be expeditiously presented to the committee for prompt necessary action. In like manner, the consultant has recourse to the committee for progress reports and presentations, contract clarification, or factors that prevent compliance with the contract. When necessary the committee may exercise its right of default and hire another consultant, or create a new contract acceptable to both parties.

The committee may involve a consultant as they *prepare* the EMS planning report, or may only require such services to *implement* the plan. The committee may request the consultant to prepare a feasibility study. This usually includes the purpose of the project, EMS program requirements for communication, the communication system design to support the EMS programs, alternate systems, physical and personnel requirements, estimated one-time and recurring costs, phase development of the communication system, conclusions, and recommendations. This phase of the study can provide the committee with data that will determine the course of action in the development of the EMS communication system.

To implement the planning, the consultant provides the engineering design of the EMS communication system, starting with a block diagram showing the kinds of communication services proposed by geographic location, interconnecting and interfacing public-safety services, other supporting agencies, and related data. With acceptance of this planning by the committee, the consultant proceeds with engineering drawings, in sufficient detail, to establish the utilization of existing equipment, alterations and additions, and specifications for procurement of additional equipment.

The consultant may provide the bidding specifications for vendors, assist in reviewing their proposals, and prepare recommendations to the committee for its acceptance or rejection. The consultant may also supervise, or oversee, the construction and installation of the communication system, evaluate the final inspection, and certify to the operational capability of the system and contract compliance. Furthermore, the consultant may assist in establishing personnel requirements for operating and maintaining the EMS communication system. This includes standards of performance and training requirements.

As the emergency medical services expand over a period of time, the consultant may return to review any changing program needs for communications, and recommend updating the system to incorporate the advantages of new technology.

This chapter has provided the reader with insight into communicating with prospective communication consultants to determine their abilities to provide the specialized engineering services needed by the EMS council to develop the EMS communication plan and follow through to the installation of an operating system.

The next chapter continues the development of the EMS communication plan by introducing the factors involved in the technical design of a basic EMS communication system. The nontechnical approach should provide the reader with a means of communicating with the technical personnel responsible for the system design and assist in evaluating the engineering recommendations on the system configuration, plan of operation, physical characteristics, and related factors.

Chapter 8

EMS Communications Equipment and System Configuration

This chapter is intended to increase the understanding by the EMS medical and management personnel of the factors involved in the technical design of a basic EMS communication system. Actually, there are more basic radio communication systems operating today in rural and small urban areas than there are complex systems in large metropolitan areas.

DESIRED SYSTEMS ATTRIBUTES

Underlying the design of the entire EMS communication system are certain general design principles. Although some may be obvious, few systems embody them all.

Accessibility and Speed: Messages must be capable of fast transmission—the system must be accessible to its users and designed to prevent costly delays. Dedicated telephone lines (control lines) or hotlines (lines reserved for a specific use), rather than public telephone service, are required for certain key communication links.

Backup: Essential communication landlines must have radio backup channels in the event of disruption of the primary links. Natural disasters can obliterate telephone and other landlines. Emergency power must be available to operate key equipment in such situations.

Compatibility: It seems likely that in the future an areawide system must be compatible with regional, state, and national EMS, disaster, and other emergency systems, including those planned for future implementation.

Continuity: Communication systems must be available for use on a 24-hour basis. Where stations in the EMS system are not staffed continuously (such as at a rural clinic or physician's office), provision must be made for alternate communication links to accomplish necessary functions during the off-duty period. Also, there must be redundancy for peak traffic capability as well as for insurance against loss of service at a critical moment.

Convenience of Use: Equipment must be simple enough to be operated easily by nontechnical people with a minimum of specific training.

Coverage: The telephone and radio systems must cover the entire geographic area. Repeater stations (radio relay devices), microwave backbone systems (a multimessage-carrying link between two or more points), and careful antenna selection and location can increase coverage.

Flexibility: The system must be flexible, maintaining the capability for efficient growth consistent with long-range projections of needs and services.

Noninterference Frequency Coordination: Radio frequencies must be carefully selected to meet the variety of EMS needs while minimizing the possibility of interference by existing users of nearby channels in the area. Frequency assignments used to communicate with other agencies must be carefully coordinated and made compatible with the agencies' operating frequencies.

Radio Spectrum Management: The competition of all users of radio communications has created an intense demand for frequency assignments with resulting congestion on the airways. Thus, radio communications should be used only where other links (such as telephone or cable) are inadequate or inefficient. Consistent with effective operations, procedures should encourage minimal use of radio facilities.

Regular Use: All communication facilities, both primary and backup, should be utilized daily to ensure their operational readiness and to keep the staff well aware of their presence and well-versed in their use.

DESIGN CONSIDERATIONS

Communication systems intended for emergency medical care require special design considerations. The major determining factors are:

1. The operational requirements of the EMS system.
2. The number and location of terminals (communication centers, hospitals, emergency medical vehicle services, clinics, and supporting agencies).
3. Topographical, geographical, and environmental considerations.
4. Quantity and sources, present or projected, of emergency calls.
5. Sophistication of EMS equipment requiring support communications, such as emergency medical vehicular equipment, paging, and telemetry.
6. Types and capabilities of existing communications equipment used in EMS systems.
7. Types and availability of physical facilities.
8. Types and availability of funding.
9. Maintaining an operational capability when public sources fail.

EQUIPMENT

Station Equipment

Before getting into communication design, some familiarity with the equipment components will be helpful. The graphics are for illustration only, and do not represent any specific brands of equipment.

Figure 8–1 has illustrations of the usual configurations of desktop base stations, which may consist of a transceiver, or a transmitter and a receiver. The microphone switch may be located on the microphone stand or on the floor; the latter frees the operator's hands for other work. Fixed base stations in upright floor racks are also shown in Figure 8–1. These racks contain the transmitter and receiver equipment. They are usually operated from a separate location, and use remote-control desk-top units (Figure 8–2). The remote-control unit amplifies the operator's voice and feeds it to the transmitter rack on a pair of wires or on a special-grade telephone cable permanently connected between the two points. The remote-control unit also uses the same cables to send an electronic signal to turn the transmitter on when keyed at the remote-control unit. this unit has the means of controlling the volume of the mobile station signal coming back on the channel from the remotely located base station. In this instance, it serves strictly as an audio amplifier for the incoming signal.

Desk Top Base Stations

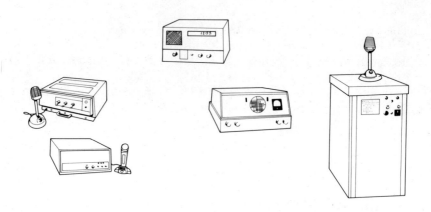

Fixed Base Station (Upright)

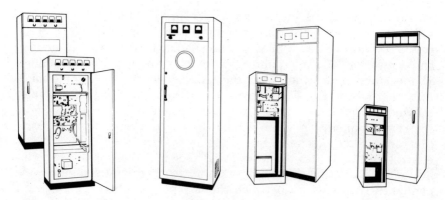

Figure 8-1. Base Station Communications Equipment.

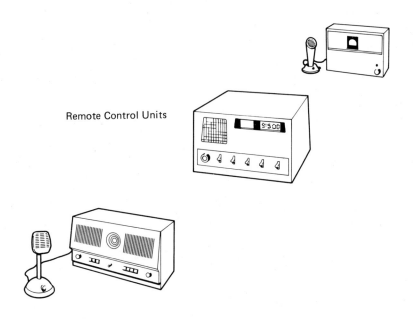

Remote Control Units

Selective Calling Units

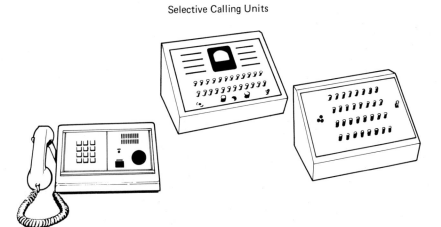

Figure 8-2. Remote Control and Selective Calling Units.

The use of floor racks to contain the radio units may be for convenience or for efficiency. High-power transmitting equipment is normally rack-mounted. Multichannel systems may use several of the floor-mounted racks.

The communication center may have one or more monitor receivers, tuned to the frequency of transmitters in the EMS communication system and to those of the public-safety agencies. These receivers are also used to cross-monitor the transmissions with another radio system; that is, each system transmits on its own channel and receives the signal of the other system on a monitor receiver, thus achieving two-way communications (See Figure 8-3).

Selective Calling

An accessory that is frequently used at the transmitter control position is a selective-calling unit (see Figure 8-2). A system so equipped can transmit to a preselected base station, mobile unit, or personal pager to the exclusion of all others.

Antennas

Some of the more commonly used base station VHF antennas for two-way radio communication are shown in Figure 8-4. Manufacturers make various versions of the three types illustrated, depending on the channel to be used and the radiation pattern desired. The omnidirectional antenna is designed to transmit and receive equally in all directions. The cardiod antenna produces a heart-shaped pattern and is frequently used near the borders of adjacent radio systems to direct the signal into the desired area and reduce signal strength in the adjacent system area, where it might cause interference. The unidirectional antenna is designed to concentrate a large amount of the signal in only one direction, with very little radiation in the opposite direction, and is often used to provide point-to-point communications for radio-control or repeater-type service. The area coverage depends upon antenna gain, height above ground, surrounding terrain, frequency being used, power output of the transmitter, and other related factors. Similar techniques are used in antennas for other channels such as UHF.

An antenna array providing a negative vertical radiation pattern may be used to radiate a signal into a valley from an outside source. This is illustrated in Figure 8-5. This antenna is designed to concentrate the radiated signal in the desired direction, and can be adjusted to provide an angle favorable to the radiation pattern wanted.

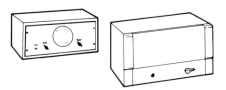

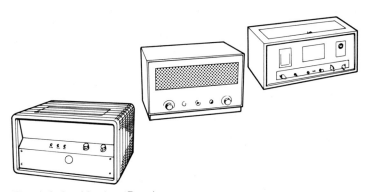

Figure 8-3. Monitor Receivers.

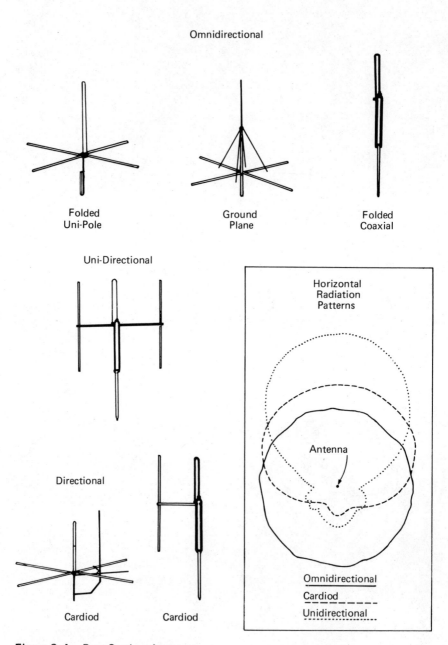

Figure 8-4. Base Station Antennas.

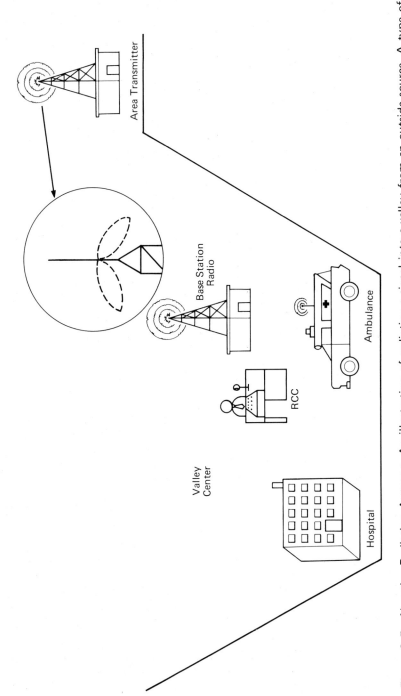

Figure 8-5. Negative Radiation Antenna. An illustration of radiating a signal into a valley from an outside source. A type of antenna with a negative radiation beam tilt is shown in the circle.

Mobile Radios

Mobile radio units are basically of the same electronic design as the base stations. They have power supplies designed for their environment. Vehicular units draw their power from the vehicle's battery. Some mobile radios are designed to operate from either the vehicle's battery or, when removed from the vehicle, from batteries contained within the radio unit itself. Mobile radios are very compact, and may be designed so that components such as the speaker and squelch- and volume-control units can either be combined with the transmitter and receiver units or separated to provide for various types of vehicle installations. Mobile radio units are limited in transmitter power output because of their limited power supply, size limitations, and antenna limitation (see Figure 8-6).

Portable Radios

Portable radio units include hand-held units and pack sets (see Figure 8-7). The portable units operate from self-contained batteries, and may be used by a person while in motion. Some units have adapters so they can be operated on 115 volts AC commercial power from a fixed location.

The hand-held portable radios have a limited range because of the limited size of the unit, batteries, and antenna. The pack sets usually have a greater power output and range.

Limitations

Portable and mobile radios have the advantage of mobility, but they have limitations. The transmitting and receiving range between the calling and receiving stations is limited by the necessary technical compromises in the equipment and by the environmental surroundings in which they operate. For portability, the size and number of batteries used for power is a limitation. This, in turn, limits the amount of power output that can be designed into the transmitter. Obviously the antenna on a portable unit must be restricted in length and type; this also reduces the transmitting and receiving range.

The surrounding buildings, hills, trees, wooded areas, and other obstructions that are in the signal path between the portable or mobile radio and other station may reflect or absorb enough of the signal to result in a weak or distorted signal, or no signal at all. Many times a better signal path can be found by changing location. Possible solutions in such a situation are to get the communication stations closer together and in a position that will circumvent the negative effects of the environment, or to use satellite receiver, or to saturate the area with a signal.

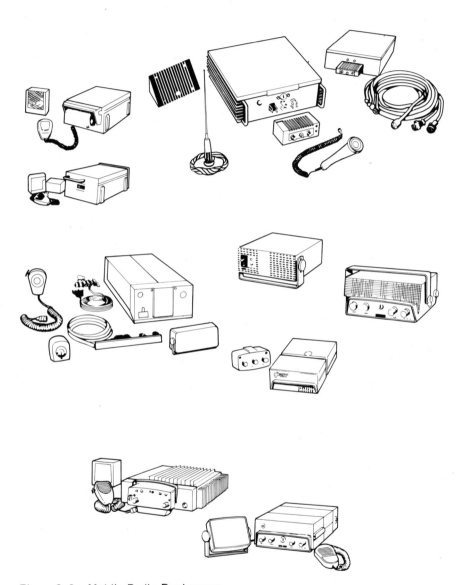

Figure 8-6. Mobile Radio Equipment.

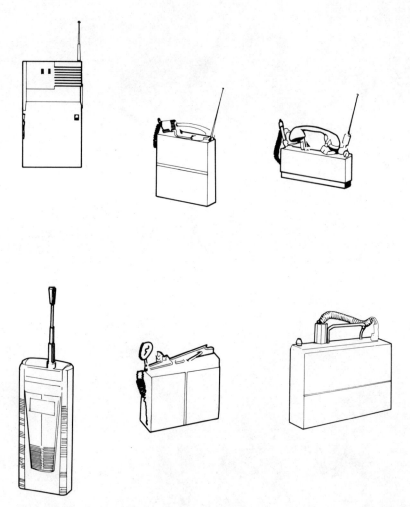

Figure 8-7. Portable Radio Units.

The Simplex System

For illustration, a radio communication system can be designed as a combination of fixed (by location) and mobile stations. Each will have a transmitter and a receiver. Each system must be licensed by the Federal Communications Commission, the agency that will assign a specific radio operating channel, or group of channels, that may be used in the system.

To understand the complexities in the design of a radio communication system, the basic simplex two-way system provides a good beginning. This is usually a single-channel system in which the base station and the mobile unit operate on the same frequency. It is a simplex system because the base station and the mobile units must transmit alternately, and the receiver is automatically silenced (muted) by the push-to-talk switch at the station performing the transmission. The transmitting operator, therefore, must release the push-to-talk switch after each transmission to hear the answering station.

The operating controls of a desk-top base station are generally located on the front panels of the radio equipment. The only controls that should be readily accessible to the operator are the receiver volume control, squelch control, and the microphone switch. The volume control is used as on any standard radio. The squelch control adjusts the receiver to mute or squelch the static noise normally present if there is no incoming radio signal. Microphones are generally provided with a push-to-talk switch mounted on the microphone as a means of turning on the transmitter and simultaneously muting the receiver.

Mobile radio units are provided with the same operating controls as the base station equipment. The controls must be located in a convenient place for the operator. A mobile installation in an ambulance will require dual control positions.

Base Stations

The design of a local control base station with the associated mobile units and accessories to a radio communication system is shown in Figure 8-8. It is the most basic system in common use today. The system is designed for a two-way radio communication between a fixed base station and mobile units in a given area. Vehicle-to-vehicle radio communication is possible when they are in sufficiently close proximity, determined in part by the terrain and the power output of the mobile radio units.

In Figure 8-8 the base station has a radio transmitter identified as T-1, a receiver as R-1, and a power supply operating from a

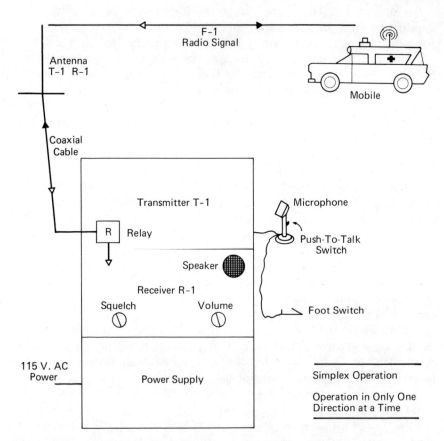

Figure 8-8. Local Control Base Station.

utility power source. These units are normally contained in one cabinet, such as the desk type. The receiver has the squelch and volume controls on the front panel within easy reach of the operator. The loudspeaker is also mounted on the front panel. The microphone is an external device equipped with a push-to-talk switch. The transmitter may also have a foot-operated switch located on the floor under the operator's desk, which frees the operator's hands for writing or other functions while operating the transmitter.

When the operator holds down the push-to-talk switch, it mutes the receiver and turns on the transmitter unit, which generates a radio signal on the channel assigned to the system by the FCC. This signal goes through the antenna-switching relay to the coaxial transmission line and in turn to the antenna, as indicated by the black arrows in Figure 8-8. The antenna is designed to operate on the same channel for maximum radiation of the radio signal, f-1. Since this is a simplex operation, the mobile radio unit will be in a receive mode except when the mobile operator is transmitting, and for this illustration, the mobile operator will receive the message from the base operator.

The transmission from the mobile radio unit is similar in operation. The radio signal from the mobile unit antenna, indicated by the white arrows in Figure 8-8, is received by the base station antenna, through the coaxial cable and switched through the relay to the receiver, R-1, where it is converted from radio frequencies to voice frequencies.

The basic information provided by this illustration will carry over in the design of more complex systems with more capabilities using additional units and accessories to meet specific EMS program requirements.

Extended Control Base Stations

Generally the operator's communication control center is located on the lower floor of the building of the agency using the communication system, such as the emergency department of a hospital. These are usually unsatisfactory locations for transmitting and receiving antennas due to surrounding obstacles or radio noise generated by nearby electrical devices. When this situation exists, the base station is usually set up at a distance from the control unit. If the antenna system can operate satisfactorily from the roof of the same building, an extended local control unit with associate control cables (see Figure 8-9) is available as an accessory. This unit contains a microphone and switch, and a unit with the necessary power switch, loudspeaker, and squelch and volume controls. They extend

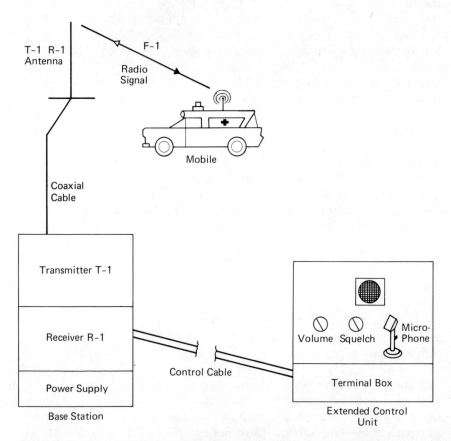

Figure 8-9. Extended Control Base Station Simplex operation. Single Frequency System.

the local control unit up to the distance limited by the manufacturer's specifications. The transmitter, receiver, relays, and power supply are rack-mounted in cabinets on an upper floor of the building near the antenna system to keep the connecting coaxial cable as short as possible.

The system design illustrated in Figure 8-9 is similar to that in Figure 8-8, except that the radio equipment is mounted in floor-type racks and located at a distance from the operator's console.

Remote Control Base Stations

If the surrounding terrain precludes use of a building roof antenna system for base-to-mobile communications, the communications design will include a remote-control base station. This remote operation of the system provides for the antenna system, base transmitter, and receiver to be located a considerable distance from the control point to take advantage of higher terrain and a noise-free area to obtain desired signal coverage. This system design is shown in Figure 8-10.

The base station equipment is essentially the same as shown for the extended remote-control center in Figure 8-9, with one exception: a remote-control unit has been included to permit remote-control operation of the base station using the telephone wire cable between the base station and the operator's remote-control center. This is necessary because of the greater distances between the base station and the remote-control center. This operator's remote-control center may be several miles from the site of the base station. The remote-control unit contains voice amplifiers, relays, power supply, and related equipment. It may be a desk-top cabinet, or floor-mount cabinet with only the necessary controls in the desk-top unit. This control unit enables the operator to turn on the base station and perform all the transmitting and receiving functions through the interconnecting telephone wire cable.

Radio Controlled Remote Base Station

The system design illustrated in Figure 8-11 shows a base station remotely controlled by radio signals in place of the telephone wire cables shown in Figure 8-10. It is used when the interconnecting telephone cables are not available, not practical, too expensive, or too vulnerable to failure. This is still a radio simplex system, even though additional stations and frequencies are used for radio control and relay purposes.

This communication system is designed to provide remote control of the base station by radio, and the use of radio-controlled relay

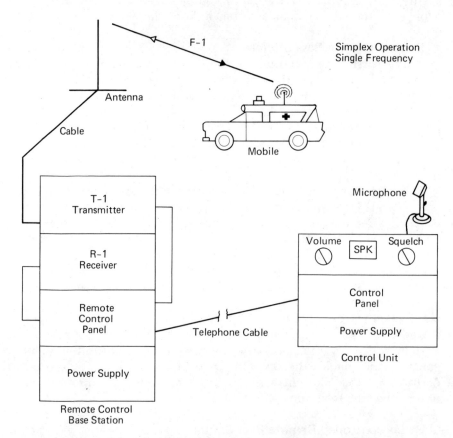

Figure 8-10. Remote Controlled Base Station. Simplex Operation Single Frequency.

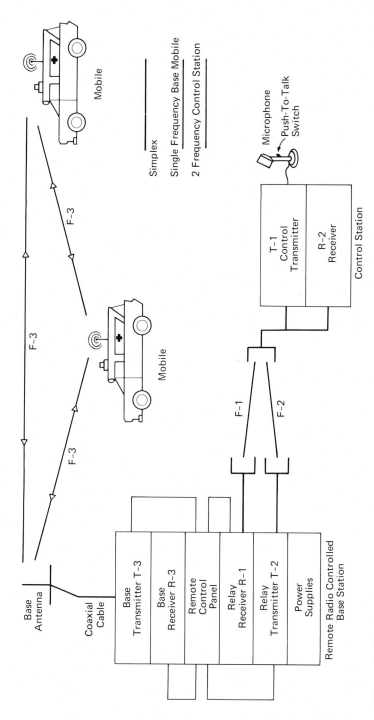

Figure 8-11. Remote Radio-Controlled Base Station.

circuits. This type of system includes a separate transmitter (T-2) and receiver (R-1) for operating the controlling circuit, in addition to the base station transmitter (T-3) and the receiver (R-3). This control equipment operates on different radio channels from the base station to prevent an undesirable interaction between their operation. It also enables the operator at the remote-control station to have control of the remote base station transmitter at all times.

The control station includes a transmitter (T-1) and receiver (R-2) with a microphone and the standard controls, and a highly directional antenna. The directional antenna is used to direct a signal from the control station transmitter (T-1) to the antenna of the remote base station control receiver (R-1) operating on the same channel (f-1). The signal coming from receiver R-1 goes through the radio-controlled panel (RCP) and automatically causes the base transmitter to turn on and retransmit the original signal on the T-3 transmitter to the receive in the emergency vehicle, which is heard by the operator.

When the operator of the emergency vehicle uses the mobile transmitter f-3 channel, this procedure is reversed. The signal received by the base station receiver (R-3) goes through the remote-controlled panel, causing the relay transmitter T-2 to turn and retransmit the signal on channel f-2 to receiver R-2 at the control station.

As this system is designed for simplex mobile operation, any of the emergency vehicles having a transmitter and receiver on the same f-3 channel may communicate with each other provided they are within range, the limiting factors being the environment and the radiation pattern of the mobile antennas.

TWO CHANNEL RADIO SYSTEMS

Although simplex systems are in common use today, it is apparent that there are certain limitations that can be detrimental in an emergency medical communication system. For example, with the simplex system, if an emergency call is made from a mobile radio or another base station to an EMS control center that is transmitting at the time, the control center receiver would be muted and the operator would not receive the call. The emergency call could not be completed until the control center had stopped transmitting. This loss of time in an EMS emergency could be critical. Therefore, many communication systems are designed for two-channel duplex operation to expedite emergency traffic.

One way to achieve duplex operation is to expand the simplex system. This design of a two-channel system is shown in Figure 8-12. The base station in this system uses the familiar single channel f-1 in conjunction with base transmitter T-1 and base receiver R-1 for base-to-mobile communications. This same channel is shared by the mobile units for vehicle-to-vehicle communications if desired. The white arrows between the base station and the mobile units indicate the simplex communications operation on the f-1 channel. The base station receiver R-1 is used to receive calls from the mobile units or to monitor mobile-to-mobile communications within the range of the base station. All operation on the f-1 channel is still simplex operation, whereby the base an the mobile receivers R-1 are muted at the station performing the transmission.

To make this a two-channel system, the design includes a base station receiver R-2, identified in Figure 8-12 as "priority channel" mobile-to-station only, and a control unit. This second receiver R-2 operates on a different frequency from receiver R-1, and is not muted when the base station is transmitting. The mobile operator can now switch the transmitter to this priority-channel frequency, f-2, as indicated by the black arrow, and be received by the base station operator even though the base station transmitter is being used. For clarity, the illustration in Figure 8-12 uses two receive antennas and one transmit antenna. In practice, only one antenna may be needed when the channel separation is sufficient and by the use of special electronic accessories.

Mobile units in this two-channel system have only one receiver and transmitter. The transmitter, however, is designed to selectively operate on either of two channels with the addition of a switching device to enable the operator to change channels. The transmitter can operate on only one channel at a time, and must be switched for operation on f-1 or f-2.

ONE-WAY TALKBACK REMOTE RECEIVER SYSTEM

Figure 8-13 shows the design of a one-way talkback radio relay system. This is an expansion of the two-channel system design shown in Figure 8-12. In this illustration the base station has a medium- to high-power transmitter. With a tower-mounted antenna of sufficient height, the station may have sufficient *talkout* power to send to mobile units located a considerable distance from the base station. The mobile unit, however, located that far away, usually does not have enough *talkback* power to send directly the base station because mobile units are limited in transmitting power by the capacity

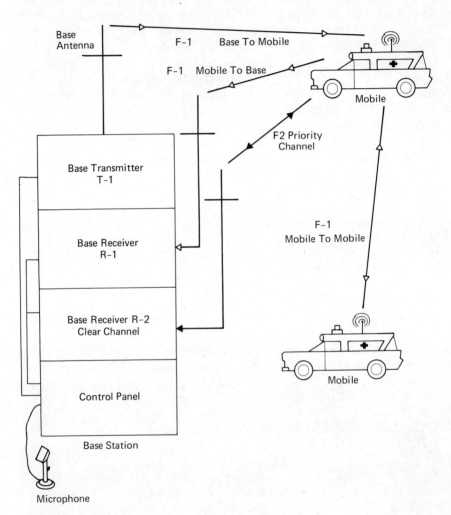

Figure 8-12. Two Frequency System.

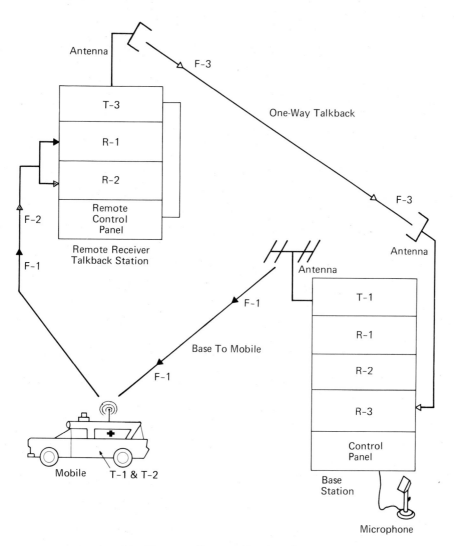

Figure 8-13. One Way Talkback Remote Receiver System.

of the vehicle battery—their source of power input—and antenna height is limited and thus less efficient.

In large areas served by a radio communication system, one or more automatic one-way talkback radio receiver stations are included to increase the talkback range of the mobile units in the system. This also enables the base station to monitor vehicle mobile-to-mobile communications at the distant areas of the system. By doing so, the operator can avoid interrupting emergency mobile-to-mobile communications.

To extend the range of the mobile transmitter, the radio system design includes a one-way talkback receiver system. In Figure 8–13 the emergency vehicle can receive the radio signal from the base station transmitter T–1, but the base station cannot receive the mobile transmissions on f–1 and f–2 because the vehicle is located too great a distance from the base station. The radio receiver station, however, is within receiving distance of the mobile radio which can transmit on frequencies f–1 and f–2. This receiver station is automatic and unattended. When its receivers R–1 and R–2 receive a signal on either channel f–1 or f–2, it automatically sends it to transmitter T–3. This transmitter repeats the message from the mobile unit and, using a highly directional antenna, sends it to the base station on frequency f–3. The base station picks up the transmission on a directional antenna and receiver R–3.

Note that the base station receiver R–3 is in addition to the two-channel equipment, that is, T–1, R–1, and R–2 for communication with mobile units within the normal range of the base station. For clarity, this capability was not duplicated on this illustration.

The f–3 channel used for this radio receiver is different from the base station and mobile unit channels to prevent interchannel interference at the remote receiver station and the base station. This makes possible a clear channel call-in type of operation from a single mobile unit to the base station through the remote receiver station.

Channels used for the automatic radio receiver stations may be in the VHF, UHF, or microwave bands. The actual channel or group of channels authorized depends upon many factors, including distances involved, terrain, and availability of channels in the assigned radio frequency area. This configuration can be expanded to include a number of locations for the remote receivers, with their signal output applied to an evaluation circuit to select the best signal to feed to the base station. This mode of operation is usually referred to as a *receiver voting system*.

INTERSYSTEM COMMUNICATIONS

With any of the two-way radio systems involved in public safety, such as the emergency medical vehicle service, hospitals, police departments, fire departments, and other agencies providing direct support, it is permissible to intercommunicate providing the information exchanged is necessary and pertains directly to the emergency, and is consistent with the primary responsibility of the licensee of the system.

Figure 8-14 shows one means of intersystem communications, known as cross-monitoring or cross-band operation. This illustration uses the single-channel simplex system for clarity, but the same principle applies to more complex systems.

As shown, the two base stations are a part of separate county EMS systems, and in times of an EMS emergency may have the need to communicate by radio. To accomplish this by cross-monitoring, each base station installs a radio receiver that is tuned to receive the signals of the other's base station transmitter.

When the base station operator in county A needs to communicate with the base station in county B, the operator uses transmitter T-1 on the same f-1 channel used to call a mobile unit in the county A. The difference is, the operator identifies the base station in county B when placing the call. The signal from county A is heard by the operator in county B on their receiver R-1. When county B answers the call, the operator transmits T-2 on their system channel f-2, and it is received by the operator in county A on their receiver R-2.

This method of two-way communication is simple and economical but the use of two single-channel radio systems in this manner *negates* all other traffic during the transmission time. Mobile units in both of the counties will hear only one side of the conversation. Where it is necessary for mobile units of each county to have intersystem communication, they may install a separate monitor receiver in the vehicle tuned to receive the other system and operate in the same manner.

The design of this simplex and two-channel radio system can be expanded, duplicated as subsystems, and when combined may be used as a complete system. The radio communication design possibilities, with the present inventory of radio hardware and accessories, is vast. The communication needs of any operating EMS system can be technically provided by the present state of the communications art. In most cases, implementing and planning requires only decision and funding.

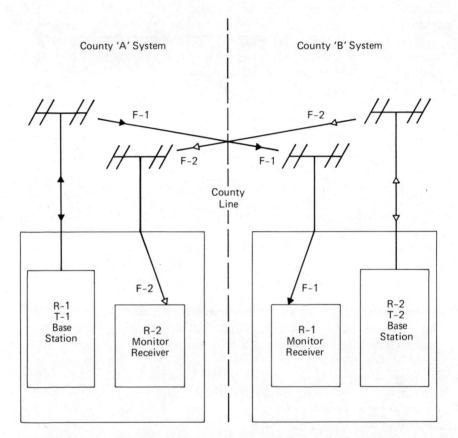

Figure 8-14.   Inter-System Communications.

SYSTEM DEVELOPMENT

Many chapters could be written on the improvements that have been made in radio communication design beyond the basic simplex and multichannel system described.

Monitoring radios have a scanning device that enables one receiver to constantly monitor many frequencies. Radio signals can transmit data in addition to voice. One such technique is identified as telemetry—a method of sensing and measuring information at a distant location and transmitting the measured data by radio signals to a central location where they are received for recording and analysis. An example is the radio transmission of an electrocardiogram (ECG) of a patient at the scene of a medical emergency by an ambulance attendant, to be received in the emergency room of a preselected hospital for analysis for an attending physician. Transmitters and receivers operate from a selection of several frequencies. Radio control center operators monitor and coordinate the operation and the use of the EMS communication system.

Expansion of the system design to include additional systems, channels, accessories, computers, and automatic devices should only be considered if: (1) the overall EMS communication system will be *measurably* improved; (2) this improvement will directly benefit the emergency medical services provided; and (3) there be an *economical* savings through more efficient utilization of available resources.

Although not exhaustive, this nontechnical discussion of a highly technical subject has provided an insight to the basic system configurations. Larger systems are multiples or combinations of basic systems with the additions of accessories to meet the requirements of individual systems.

Once the system design is firm, the next step, Chapter 9, concerns the preparation of the operational and technical specifications that are prepared for inclusion in bid proposals the buyer sends to appropriate vendors.

Chapter 9

Specifications

The consultant or engineer will establish the technical specifications for the equipment to be procured for the EMS communication system. These specifications involve all aspects of the equipment, including the state of the art, technical circuitry, tolerances, operational capability, operating controls, physical size, weight, environmental requirements, maintenance contracts and availability of service, flexibility of operation, and adaptability to expansion of the system.

GENERAL CONSIDERATIONS

The technical specifications for the equipment should provide a system having the maximum state-of-the-art capability, as well as time-saving operations with minimum personnel requirements. In some instances, however, there may be constraints. The system being assembled may be a subsystem of an existing public-safety system, and the design specifications will be for equipment that is compatible with this existing system. Even when circumstances dictate a minimum, no-frills, basic system or subsystem, the specifications should allow for eventual expansion.

The design specifications include the physical characteristics required of the installation. No two need be alike. However, the engineer drawing up the specifications, the personnel who provide the space for the communications equipment, and the personnel who will be operating the equipment must agree on the physical characteristics of the equipment to be involved.

Building space available and suitable for installation of racks of equipment must be located and dedicated to this service. One consideration is the relationship between components, for some units must be located close to one another while others can be a greater distance apart without a sacrifice in efficiency. Other considerations include the weight distribution, floor space for installation, and access space for servicing, ventilation, temperature extremes, humidity, a dust-free environment, and security.

Antennas must be located in an area that will provide the required radiation pattern. The type of antenna, supporting superstructure, and geographic location are selected so that the combination will provide the maximum radio signal necessary to the appropriate radio equipment.

The tower base, whether on the roof of a building or on the ground, must be sufficient to support the antenna superstructure and guy wires (if used). Depending on the type of antenna and transmitter/receiver equipment, the proximity of the two must be within the technical limitation.

Physical considerations for the location of the control console include the size, weight, and convenience to the operating and maintenance personnel. Environmental considerations are noise, contaminants, temperature extremes, humidity, ventilation, and security.

The technical circuitry of the proposed system should conform to current engineering practices. Operational tolerances of the hardware items may vary between vendors, and the requirements must be determined by the engineer designing the system. Considerations include such constraints as the radio channels assigned by the FCC, antenna sites, frequency interference from adjoining systems, and the complexity of the system design.

The mechanical features of the hardware items also vary among vendors. Some mobile units have from four to ten pushbuttons plus knobs for the driver to manipulate. The specifications should provide for maximum simplicity in operation, consistent with the system objectives. Operating procedures and controls should be sufficiently simple and standardized to assure proper operation of the system even when the personnel assigned to this task are operating under stress. A degree of ruggedness is required for dependability when the equipment is operated by several different people with various degrees of dexterity and operating skills.

When there are multiple base and mobile stations in the system, a tone-coded squelch system is advantageous. Mobile transmitter receivers in emergency medical vehicles must have an extended control to permit operation from the patient compartment.

The specifications for the operational capacity of the basic hardware items should provide for the immediate needs of the system, as well as for future expansion. This capacity for expansion may be in the form of accessories that provide automation, additional functions, or relieve operators of mechanical functions. There may be an expansion of the circuitry within the hardware units to accommodate additional channels. An increase in the number of mobile stations should be accommodated by the communication control center through the use of additional units of equipment, or have an expansion capability to accommodate an additional dispatcher.

Reliability is most important in an EMS communication system and should be a primary factor when evaluating components and subsystems, both new and existing. Vendors normally perform reliability engineering studies and tests; this data should be available for comparative purposes.

CATEGORIES OF SPECIFICATIONS

Bid specifications for a radio communications system are usually in one of three categories, as detailed below.

The Specified System

In a *specified* system, the consultant is responsible for the design, detailed drawings, wiring diagrams, and specifications for each item of hardware. The consultant also determines the antenna design for specific coverage, the radio relay station survey, the compatibility of physical facilities; directs the installation; performs all acceptance testing; and assumes responsibility for operation. Furthermore the consultant prepares the application for FCC licensing and frequency assignment.

Specifications for hardware items can be tailored to meet design requirements that may be difficult to obtain from off-the-shelf items of major suppliers. A survey of suppliers will identify those with the capacity to provide or custom-build the needed items. Separate bid specifications are prepared on each item. The accepted bids may provide a heterogeneous combination of brands working together. Their compatibility depends on the accuracy of the design specifications, tolerances of the delivered item, and the efficiency of the design.

The Turnkey Method

In the turnkey method a contract is made with one vendor to design, install, and be fully responsible for the successful operation and maintenance of the system for a specified period of time. These contracts are usually awarded through competitive bidding, and are sometimes known as guaranteed performance contracts.

The EMS council or agency using the turnkey method provides the desired performance specifications in their bid proposal. These are based on the EMS communication planning report, and the consultant's or engineer's technical recommendations. The extent of the specifications depends upon the desired sophistication. Important considerations include:

1. The limits of the EMS catchment area requiring guaranteed radio coverage, shown on suitable geographical and topographical maps.
2. The extent and nature of the network of base and mobile stations and portable units to be served by the RCC.
3. A system design, based on engineering surveys, to ensure minimum intermodulation and interference. If point-to-point microwave links are to be built at a later time, consideration must be given to compatibility and minimum interference.
4. Mobile units must be able to maintain continuous communication, directly or by relays, with other units or base stations located within the designated area. This may require a voting capability in conjunction with the relays. This should include tone-coded squelch.
5. A block diagram of the contractor design, including the engineering features, radio channels, signal paths, base station and relay locations, commercial and emergency power requirements, and related data.
6. If the system is to be integrated with existing VHF equipment, this must be clearly identified in the block diagram with the engineering features. Modifications to the existing design and equipment must be clearly defined by drawings and text.
7. Hospital paging will be separate and designed to meet the requirements established in the EMS communications planning report.
8. Solid-state electronic equipment is preferable, using the latest state-of-the-art design.
9. The terms of the maintenance contract must clearly identify the agency that will perform the maintenance, the extent of the service, and the period of time.
10. The vendor's plan for the phased integration of the new with the old system, when applicable to the project, must be included.
11. There must be an expansion capability with a minimum of equipment replacement.
12. The vendor must provide a description of the tests to be

performed, the results to be observed, test equipment they will use, number of personnel, and amount of time to perform the acceptance testing.

13. The vendor must provide a plan for dispatcher operational training and for maintenance personnel schooling prior to activation of the communication system.

The Combination Method

The combination method is a *compromise* between the preceding two. The specifications are written in individual contracts for the electronic hardware, wiring, installation, and the non-electronic construction. This enables the EMS council or agency to use the in-house capability of the organization to perform as many of the tasks as practical and economical. The consultant or engineer supervises the individual contracts and the integration of the several parts to an operating communication system.

Summary

Each method has advantages. The specific method is claimed to be more economical than the turnkey, but only if the engineering expertise is available in-house. Another plus claimed is the ability to procure nearly custom-designed hardware items. Maintenance after the guarantee can be more complex depending on the number of different brands of equipment being serviced.

The turnkey method can be very effective with a guaranteed operation. The expertise required for the final design and specifications is shifted to the vendor. The design will normally utilize the vendor's products and, because of the guarantee clause in the contract, the vendor will be more inclined to overbuild than to underbuild. This method should be predominantly from one manufacturer, which may limit the design but could simplify maintenance.

The combination method is in common practice and, where applicable, may provide an economical approach to the contract funding through the combination of in-house capabilities and competitive bidding.

In the final analysis, the consultant and engineering services are paid by separate contract, or by other accounts if they are in-house employees. The expertise must be provided, no matter which method is used.

There are many more specifications that may be considered, depending on the requirements established in the planning report, such as additional encoder/decoder requirements, mobile relay equipment, need for telemetry, mobile touch-tone decoders, automatic mobile identification, and related accessories. And there are nonelectronic specifications for the base station consoles, mechanical operations, tower construction, equipment housing, and related items.

CONTRACT FORMS

Contracts generally follow the dictates of the attorneys representing the EMS council or agency concerned. The first part of the contract is often called "boilerplate," and concerns the legal aspects for both parties. It provides the means of recourse in the event of the failure of either party to meet the terms of the contract. These terms include such items as time schedules, allowable variances, insurance, surety bonds, compliance with local, state, and federal regulations, penalties, and related matters.

The equipment and performance specifications that are a part of the contract must be understood by both parties. To provide some assurance of this understanding, a prebid conference of interested vendors and the EMS council representatives can be held to review, item by item, the specifications and terms of the proposed bid and contract. This provides the vendors with an opportunity to discuss, question, and rebut prior to issuance of the invitation to bid.

A format should be prescribed for bids submitted by the vendors. This consistency in bid submissions will assist in evaluating like items during the review.

BID REVIEW

The bids submitted by the vendors should first be reviewed by the EMS council attorney for legal compliance. Then the consultant or engineer accepts those that have been approved by the legal staff and reviews the specifications of each bid submitted for the basic compliance, plus any additional capability and service the bidder included. The results of these reviews are documented, identifying the advantages and disadvantages of each. They may also be identified in numerical order indicating each reviewer's preference. The final decision, however, is made by the council representing the participants in the EMS system.

CONTRACTOR PERFORMANCE

When the successful vendor delivers the equipment and makes the installation, each completed function is inspected by the engineer representing the council. Usually, as a part of the contract, the vendor provides the equipment and personnel to demonstrate that the operation of the equipment as a system meets or exceeds all specifications. Evaluation of this demonstration is made by the consultant or engineer and recorded in a report to the EMS council, recommending acceptance of the system as meeting the terms of the contract or identifying variances that must be corrected before there can be an acceptance. When the vendor claims to have corrected any variances, the process is repeated until there is an acceptance, or the variances are reported to the legal staff for necessary action.

This chapter has provided the many technical and planning considerations that need to be resolved prior to contract negotiation. The chapter concludes with the final steps of bidding and contractual procedures that may be used, with appropriate safeguards, and concludes with the contract negotiation for procurement of the system equipment, installation, and operation.

The final Chapter 10 summarizes the preceding chapters, with emphasis on the sequence of events necessary in EMS communications planning, and the rationale of the authors in arriving at this sequence.

Chapter 10

Summary

The objective of this book, as stated in Chapter 1, is to provide noncommunication personnel involved in developing regional emergency medical services systems with a general understanding of the application, design, and implementation of a supporting EMS communication system. The book is divided into two parts. The first part develops a study and evaluation of present and future EMS objectives and the present operational procedures used in the system programs. The second part, using the findings generated in the first, develops the requirements for this resource—communications—to improve the operational capabilities of existing EMS programs and to project future requirements.

It is readily apparent that such a study involves more professional personnel than communication engineers, even though the end result is a communication system. Chapter 2 identifies the seven sequential functions involved in the operation of an EMS system. Each element is expanded to provide data on operational details that are necessary considerations in developing a supporting communication system. The role of resource management is examined in terms of their development of the several programs and agencies into a homogeneous, coordinated EMS system. These include public education, personnel training, medical direction, expansion, and related parameters of an EMS system.

To prepare a study that will identify these functions as they apply to a specific EMS system, a group of professional and lay personnel are selected to form an EMS council, as explained in Chapter 3. The talents of these individuals are identified, and an organizational chart and committee objectives are provided. This council becomes the spearhead for developing the regional EMS system whose end product is an EMS planning report that evaluates the present EMS system, develops corrective actions, and plans for future expansion. This plan is the basis for all actions that are to follow.

The techniques of developing an EMS planning report, as described in Chapter 3, are designed to provide the medical and management staff with an evaluation of their EMS system and to identify those functions that require communications. A large amount of detail is provided because the effectiveness of all communication system planning and operational procedures is based on the thoroughness and accuracy of this report. The EMS council members must be carefully selected, the analysis of the system complete, and the report an accurate evaluation.

When the EMS planning report is completed and the findings and objectives agreed on by the EMS council, the report becomes the basis for developing the second part of the book, a comprehensive EMS communication plan for the EMS system. As a prelude to this task, Chapter 5 is a nontechnical explanation of the capabilities of EMS communication systems. It is designed to provide the EMS council and staff members with a basic understanding of the many services communication can provide in support of EMS programs.

Chapter 6, building on the previous chapters, provides the basic considerations in developing an EMS communication plan. These are applied in developing specific system and equipment configurations for the EMS communication plan. At this point, the EMS council should include the services of a communication engineer knowledgeable in the design of EMS communication systems, the development of system and equipment specifications, contract negotiation, and system acceptance testing. Whether selecting a person from the in-house staff or hiring from an outside source, Chapter 7 is beneficial to identifying the required services, conducting the interview, evaluating proposals, determining contract requirements, and selecting a project director.

Recapping, through the activities of the EMS council, an EMS planning report is created. It is the basis for present and projected operation of the EMS system, a basic understanding of EMS communications, and the development of an EMS communication plan. An EMS communication engineer is on the council or a consultant has been hired to provide the necessary technical assistance. To further the development of the EMS communication plan, Chapter 8 includes design considerations and types of equipment and develops basic EMS communication system for the EMS communication plan.

Once the EMS council has agreed to the communication system design, the engineering specifications are developed preparatory to submitting requests for bids from vendors. These bids are reviewed by the EMS council and engineering advisors. The installation by the selected vendor is monitored by representatives of the EMS council and a communication engineer to assure there is contract compliance and the system provides the planned operational performance.

This completes the sequence of events in developing an EMS communication system. It starts with an evaluation of the EMS system and concludes with a communication system that provides support to the individual EMS program and the integrated EMS system. Through a basic understanding, the medical staff and the communication engineer have combined their talents to produce the most needed resource in the EMS system—a functional communication system.

Additional information on the Federal Communications Commission rules and regulations that concern EMS communications is found in Appendix A, and funding information appears in Appendix B. Reading references and a glossary of terms complete the book.

Appendix A

The Federal Communications Commission and EMS

The transmission of radio signals and their satisfactory reception has become a part of everyone's life and accepted as a matter of fact. But during the past few years we have become aware of the limitations of this resource. The presently known limitations of the radio spectrum have necessitated the establishment of controls to provide the greatest number of services to the most people requiring access to radio communications.

Since radio frequency propagation does not recognize man-made artificial boundaries, it was necessary to establish worldwide controls by international treaty. Within the United States, the Interdepartmental Radio Advisory Committee (IRAC) is responsible for the coordination and assignment of radio frequencies used by federal government agencies. The Communications Act of 1934 established the Federal Communications Commission (FCC) to encourage the effective use of nongovernment radio in the public interest.

The FCC, by statute, is charged with developing the efficient use of the radio spectrum. In practical terms, the goal is to provide rules that promote the orderly use of radio facilities and the radio frequency spectrum by the maximum number of persons. To accomplish that goal, the FCC has promulgated various rules with which licensees must comply.

When a change in regulations is contemplated, the FCC issues a "Notice of Inquiry and Rule Making" and assigns a docket number to the proposed rule. Prior to the final issuance of this notice as a "Report and Order," the public and organizations affected by the decision have time in which to express their opinions on the matter, which the FCC, in turn, may deny or accept. When the FCC believes they have adequately taken into account the reactions to their proposal, the "Report and Order" is published with the docket number, and becomes law. There are penalties for noncompliance.

Many of the changes and additions made to the FCC rules and regulations are the result of technical advancement in electronic communications equipment. The greatest motivating factor is the requests from the public and agencies for the assignment of more and more radio frequencies and special applications to meet the communication needs of new and expanding public and private programs, of which EMS is one. Improved technolgoy has made possible the expansion of the useable radio spectrum to provide more transmitting frequencies, and has also made it possible to crowd the useable transmitting frequencies closer together and thus increase the number of frequencies available in a given area of the radio spectrum. To take advantage of these technical advances, new rules and regulations are published by the FCC that may require existing equipment to be modified or replaced. When such rules and regulations require phasing out of older equipment and a large expenditure of funds for new equipment, the timetable for compliance may extend from one to several years.

Some changes in the rules and regulations are made as a result of frequency-utilization studies of user agencies. This may result in the shifting of radio frequency assignments for better use of this limited resource by agencies having the greatest need. Such changes in the rules and regulations may become effective in a relatively short period of time. Other changes to the rules and regulations may be initiated by public or private organizations, relative to the allocation of frequencies, utilization of frequencies for special purposes, or the regulation of operational practices.

Not all frequencies in the radio spectrum are available solely for U.S. users. These frequencies are shared worldwide. We share many radio frequencies with our Canadian and Mexican neighbors. An international coordinating committee meets periodically to determine worldwide assignments of frequencies, sharing procedures to be used, and to resolve area problems.

SHARING RADIO FREQUENCIES

Sharing of radio frequencies is a required practice in the United States. When there is sufficient distance between two or more stations and the transmitting power and direction is properly controlled, the radio stations may transmit on or near the same frequency and in the same mode without interfering with one another. There are many technical considerations and engineering principles applied in creating radio systems that simultaneously operate on or near the same frequency. For instance, TV channel numbers are duplicated in cities across the nation, but the cities are far enough apart and transmission sufficiently controlled to prevent primary interference with one another.

In some agencies, time-sharing provides a means for multiple use of a frequency. The hours during which each agency has access to the frequency are mutually arranged and agreed to by the FCC. Adjustments of transmitting power between day and night periods is often used to solve adjacent area interference problems.

GROUP LICENSING

Several FCC *Services** have been established as a means of grouping the licensees that have a commonality to their communication activities. Each of these services is assigned a specific number of frequencies in designated areas of the radio spectrum. Applicants for licenses apply for a specific frequency within a service that is applicable to their business or operational needs. Problems arise in this procedure when there are a large number of applicants in a given service for a limited number of frequencies.

Prior to the recent issue of a series of "Report and Order" dockets, the radio frequencies for agencies providing the public with emergency medical services have been included in the VHF band of the Special Emergency Radio Service (public-safety service) that are shared with nonmedical activities and interspersed with the allocations to other public-safety agencies. This radio service is intended for use by independently operating agencies having a minimal demand for a radio system and involving a minimum of capital investment in equipment and personnel. This pattern of limited communication requirements is not realistic for the immediate and future needs of EMS programs servicing the public.

In recognition of the need for an updating of the licensing and regulations to better accommodate the nation's expanding and changing requirements for medical radio service communications, the FCC determined it to be in the public interest to issue a series of dockets that would amend selected sections of the commission's rules and establish a separate service category with dedicated EMS frequencies.

---

*The general categories of the FCC Services include broadcast, aviation, marine, public safety, industrial, land transportation; amateur, citizens, disaster, and experimental; and common carrier. For specific information, contact your nearest FCC Field Engineering Office or the FCC headquarters, Washington, D.C.

UHF COMMUNICATIONS

FCC Docket No. 19880

One recent FCC docket that affects the emergency medical service communications field is Docket No. 19880 entitled "Medical Communications Services." This docket amends selected parts of the FCC's rules.[11] The summary of this docket states that these new rules provide for the establishment of a medical services category in the Special Emergency Radio Service. This category authorizes the licensing and operation of medical radio communication systems for the rendition and delivery of medical care to the public. Hospitals, ambulance companies, and physicians are eligible to apply under this category, as well as public health organizations, nursing homes, institutions, and organizations that regularly provide medical services.

The additional frequencies are primarily in the UHF band. The FCC emphasizes the flexibility of the types of communication now allowed on these frequencies by identifying the primary and secondary uses permitted to meet different requirements in specific areas. Allocations are made in paired frequencies for duplex operation. Two frequency pairs are allocated for dispatch and common-calling or mutual-aid communications; three frequency pairs primarily for biomedical telemetry operations and, secondarily, for other medical requirements; five frequency pairs are available primarily for general medical requirements and, secondarily, for telemetry and other medical or medically related communications; and four frequencies for extended portable operations in telemetry systems. These latter four frequencies are shared with the highway call box system.

It must be emphasized that these UHF frequencies that are to be used in the medical services are shared by all of the licensees in an operating area. It is the expectation of the FCC that an efficient and effective use of these new frequencies in the UHF band will be achieved by cooperation among the users in the development of a common communication system having a central dispatch and control center for the coordination of all EMS operations under an areawide communications plan. The *common communication system approach* for all of the area users promotes full capacity operations and is emphasized and encouraged in the new rules.

Changes effected in Docket No. 19880 replace the previous fragmented structure for medical communications with a more unified and comprehensive medical radio service category in the FCC's rules, largely through allocation of frequencies in the UHF band. The FCC does not contemplate that licensees of present EMS communication systems operating in the VHF band will be required to change the radio frequencies they are now using. It is believed, however, that the advantages of being a part of an areawide consolidated communication system will encourage the change.

One of the features of the new medical communications services is the FCC requirement for *coordination* of radio frequency assignments among the users in a given area. This replaces the previous requirement of *cooperation*. To share efficiently and effectively the EMS frequencies requires coordination of activities between all of the EMS agencies operating in a given area. As a result of this coordination, an areawide EMS operational plan is written and agreed upon by all participating agencies. This coordination applies to the standardization of emergency medical vehicle equipment, standards for hospital emergency departments, disaster planning, and the kinds and uses of communications.

The FCC will assist in the coordination of radio communication operations for the EMS systems. A provision of Docket 19880 states that any communication plans that are voluntarily submitted to the FCC for EMS systems will be made available for public inspection at the FCC headquarters in Washington, D.C. or Park Ridge, Illinois. The value of these plans being in the files of the FCC is to so advise applicants for a station license in areas that have filed a plan. This will help the applicants to ensure that their proposed communications operation will be compatible with the existing plan. The cover sheet for these plans submitted to the FCC is to include the area of proposed operation (county, state, region), mode of operation (VHF, UHF, biotelemetry, and the like), proposed starting date, existing systems and authorizations, names, addresses, and telephone numbers of persons to be contacted for information about the plan, or for copies of the plan.

VHF COMMUNICATIONS

Most of the present EMS radio communications are in the VHF band and will continue to be for some time. Many of these systems are providing satisfactory service for the agencies they are serving. Although the systems are limited, they are effective for the parameters of the EMS system now being served.* Others may want to take ad-

---

*To this end, the present VHF allocations for one-way medical paging systems are being retained and augmented by three additional frequencies for this use. Mobile relay operations, however, are precluded from operating in the VHF special Emergency Radio Service Category, except as required to crossband UHF and VHF medical communications systems.

vantage of the changes in the FCC rules and regulations, but need to amortize their investment in the present system before procuring new communication equipment. Recognizing that this status will remain for a considerable period of time, the FCC has adopted a number of rule changes to improve the EMS communication capability of those operating in the VHF band.

MEDICAL PAGING

Docket No. 19643 [11]

There are presently four VHF band channels that will remain available for one-way hospital paging. ECC Docket No.19643 allocates an additional three frequencies in the VHF Special Emergency Radio Service for medical paging systems in hospitals. One frequency is to be used for a limited-area, low-power, one-way paging system. The other two frequencies are allocated for wide-area paging operations. Any additional frequencies now in use for paging may continue to operate until January 1, 1980, providing they are not causing harmful interference to other two-way voice operations.

LICENSEES

Docket No. 19576 [11]

FCC Docket No. 19576 expands the categories of licensees who regularly provide or coordinate communications for the rendition and delivery of medical services to the public. These include any institutions and organizations that normally provide medical services in clinics, comprehensive public health facilities, and similar establishments.

CHANNEL FREQUENCY AUTHORIZATIONS

Under the FCC rules and regulations as applied to the emergency medical services, many additional radio channel frequencies are authorized. The following are the allocations and their specified uses:

150.775 MHZ for Handie Talkies—maximum 2.5 Watts
150.790 MHZ for Handie Talkies—maximum 2.5 Watts
These frequencies may be authorized only for voice transmissions from a portable (hand-held) unit, that is not airborne, to an emergency medical service vehicle for automatic retransmission by a repeater on a regular mobile frequency.

The following VHF frequencies are now being licensed for wide-area, one-way paging without power limitations. Voice paging on all two-way voice frequencies will be eliminated after January 1, 1980:

152.0075 MHz
163.250 MHz
 35.64 MHz
 35.68 MHz
 43.64 MHz
 43.68 MHz

The following frequency is for local area, low-power paging:

157.450 MHz—maximum 30 Watts

FCC Docket No. 19880

Docket No. 19880, effective August 15, 1974, assigned the following frequencies for EMS. In each pair, the lower frequency is assigned for base and mobile service, and the higher frequency for mobile only:

463.000/468.000 MHz (med one)
463.025/468.025 MHz (med two)
463.050/468.050 MHz (med three)
463.075/468.075 MHz (med four)
463.100/468.100 MHz (med five)
463.125/468.125 MHz (med six)
463.150/468.150 MHz (med seven)
463.175/468.175 MHz (med eight)

The first three frequency pairs thus assigned are primarily authorized for use under FCC Rule 89.503(a) for operations in biomedical telemetry systems. On a secondary basis, subject to noninterference with these systems, the frequencies may be used for any other permissible communications consistent with FCC Rule 89.503(d).

The last five pairs of frequencies are the primary working channels for the new Emergency Medical Radio Service. The primary use is for communications between medical facilities, EMS vehicles, and personnel related to medical supervision and instruction for treatment and transport of patients in the rendering or delivery of medical services, as authorized by FCC Rule 89.503(a). To provide additional system capabilities on a secondary basis, subject to noninterference to the foregoing operations, these frequencies may be utilized for any permissible communications consistent with FCC Rule 89.503(d), including biomedical telemetry transmission. Additionally, type f-2, f-3, and f-9 transmissions* may be authorized.

---

*This is a classification designator given modes of radio transmissions and adopted by international agreement. See [10].

Four frequencies are authorized for use under FCC Rules 89.503(a) for telemetry or voice transmission with a maximum transmitter output power of 1 watt from a portable telemetering unit to an emergency medical service vehicle for automatic retransmission to a hospital or other medical facility:

458.025 MHz 1 watt Portable, Voice or Telemetry
458.075 MHz 1 watt Portable, Voice or Telemetry
458.125 MHz 1 watt Portable, Voice or Telemetry
458.175 MHz 1 watt Portable, Voice or Telemetry

These frequencies are also available in the FCC local government radio service for highway radio call box operations.

FCC Docket No. 20484, effective March 15, 1976, assigns 462.950/467.950 MHz and 462.975/467.975 MHz, formerly used in police service, to medical communications services (replacing 460.525/465.525 and 460.550/465.550 MHz).

FCC LICENSING

The licensing and operation of radio stations and communication systems are regulated by the FCC according to the provisions of the Federal Communications Act of 1934, as amended. The provisions for system design and licensing that most directly concern the development of an emergency medical resource management communication system are contained in subpart P of Part 89, Volume V of the *FCC Rules and Regulations.*

All radio communication installations to be used in the EMS channels must be licensed during construction and testing and prior to being placed in operations. The Communications Act of 1934 prohibits unauthorized transmissions and provides violators with a possible maximum fine of $10,000, or a maximum of two years imprisonment, or both.

THE CLIENT AND THE CONSULTANT

These FCC rulings concerning EMS communications are intended to improve their communication capability and better serve the needs of the EMS system. Change is always questioned. Very seldom will a sweeping change be acceptable to everyone. A ruling for the majority of the users may not be entirely applicable, or may be adverse, to a minority. This is an example of where the communication consultant may serve by representing the client in obtaining the necessary exception from an FCC ruling to assure retention or development of an EMS communication system that can best serve the needs of the area served.

Appendix B

Funding

Funding for development of communication systems within states, regions, or local governments is usually single function oriented. For example, educational funds must be wholly spent for educational system activities; rural agriculture data for agriculture uses only; law enforcement funds for enforcement system activities; medical service funds for medical activities, etc.

The establishment of the Federal Inter-Agency EMS committee under the authority of the Emergency Medical Service Act of 1973 appeared to encourage share-cost of community and regional communication systems. However, most federal support available for development of communication systems or operating services are still single function oriented. There is not available, in one package, federal assistance for the development of a total emergency services communication system that can meet single agency needs on a joint-use basis and thereby effect savings. Consequently, the present federal funding sources encourage local governments to proliferate the development of independent systems that are generally uneconomical. It remains a responsibility of local and regional developers as well as EMS councils to bring together available funds and establish an acceptable formula for cost sharing of the EMS communications.

A publication entitled Federal Assistance for EMS was published in June 1975 by the Leonard David Institute of Health Economics, University of Pennsylvania. With their permission, the following pages (B-1 through B-9) from that publication have been reprinted to assist the reader in identifying the Federal agencies and the type of program they finanacially support. It also serves to emphasize the potential and importance for the EMS councils to investigate not only the present expenditures (hardware, personnel, facilities, training programs, etc.) but other possible state and local funding which may support the EMS program.

To reach any of the federal agencies regarding application for funding of an EMS program, contact the nearest Federal Information Center for the current address and telephone number of the agency. The Federal Information Center telephone number may be located in the white pages of the telephone directory under United States Government.

Table B-1. Program Guide: Index to Federal Programs

Overall Emerg. Med. System	EMS Planning	Training	Communications	Transportation	Emergency Dept.
10.423	12.302	10.423	12.305	12.305	13.228
12.308	12.309	13.284	12.319	12.321	13.235
12.315	14.702	13.305	12.321	12.X01	13.240
12.322		13.493	16.502	13.228	13.251
13.224		13.498	20.600	13.714	13.261
13.226		17.228		13.801	13.714
13.228		64.003		20.600	13.800
13.284				59.X01	13.801
13.285				64.011	14.128
14.701					59.X01
23.004					64.018

Note:

The Federal Domestic Assistance Catalog (FDAC) numbers in the six columns on this page are grouped by subject to expedite research, and correspond with the numbers in the first columns of the following pages.

Table B-2. Master Matrix: EMS–Related Federal Programs

Number/ Title	Federal Agency	Objectives Uses	Type of Assistance	Applicant Eligibility	Beneficiary Eligibility	General Program Obligations	Program Accomplishments	EMS Subsystems
10.423 Community Facilities Loans	Farmers Home Administration Dept. of Agriculture	Loans for capital and start-up expenses for rural community development (including EMS)	Guaranteed/ insured loans	Public and quasi-public associations that 1) are nonprofit; 2) have legal authority to operate facilities and to repay loans; and 3) are unable to finance project from own resources or to obtain reasonable commercial credit rates.	Same as applicant; Associations that serve residents of rural areas having populations of not more than 10,000	(Loans) FY 73: $0 FY 74: est. $ 50,000,000 FY 75: est. $200,000,000	Not applicable new program	All (including training
12.302 Civil Defense-Community Preparedness	Defense Civil Preparedness Agency DOD	Plan phases of civil defense, gain public support volunteers	Advisory services and counselling; Direct Technical Assistance	CD Directors; Gov't. Officials; Organization leaders	Same as applicant	(Salaries and expenses) Not separately identifiable	FY '73: 40,000 Publications distributed to state and local civil defense units	Emergency planning and operations in all phases of civil defense and industrial health
12.305 Civil Defense-Emergency Operating Centers (EOC)	Defense Civil Preparedness Agency DOD	Civil defense facilities to coordinate EMS activities	Project Grants	State or Local Civil Defense organizations through state Civil Defense agencies	Same as applicant	(Grants) FY '73: $6,976,375 FY '74: est. $6,500,000 FY '75: est. $6,000,000	FY '73: Federal matching funds for 452 EOC's	Facilities for coordination of EMS activities. Emergency type equipment pumps, generators, storage tanks

Table B-2. continued

Number/Title	Federal Agency	Objectives Uses	Type of Assistance	Applicant Eligibility	Beneficiary Eligibility	General Program Obligations	Program Accomplishments	EMS Subsystems
12.308 Civil Defense-Public Surplus Personal Property Donations (Surplus Property Program)	Defense Civil Preparedness Agency DOD	Donation of Federal surplus property to aid civil defense administration and operations.	Sale, Exchange, or Donation of Property and Goods	State and local civil defense organizations	Same as applicant	(Value of property donated-original acquisition cost) FY '73: $64,406,000 FY '74: est. $90,000,000 FY '75: est. $100,000,000	FY 73: 50 state participation; donations of Federal surplus personnel property	Property donation for C.D. use
12.309 Civil Defense-Industrial Participation	Defense Civil Preparedness Agency DOD	Develop facility plans and organization to survive natural or industrial disaster	Direct Technical Assistance Training	Person representing business, industry, gov't. facilities, etc.	Same as applicant	(Salaries and expenses) FY '73: $100,000 FY '74: est. $60,000 FY '75: est. $60,000	FY 73: Distributed 250,000 copies of publications; conducted three 1 week courses on industry defense	Direct Technical Assistance to develop facility plans and organization; Publications
12.315 Civil Defense-Personnel and Administrative Expenses	Defense Civil Preparedness Agency DOD	Funds to coordinate EMS activities in a disaster	Formula Grants (Matching funds)	State and local C.D. organizations	Same as applicant	(Grants) FY '73: $24,755,000 FY '74: est. $27,200,000 FY '75: est. $28,600,000	FY '73: 50 state participation; matching funds for 6,000 positions	Salaries for CD employees

125

Table B-2. continued

Number/ Title	Federal Agency	Objectives Uses	Type of Assistance	Applicant Eligibility	Beneficiary Eligibility	General Program Obligations	Program Accomplishments	EMS Subsystem
12.319 Civil Defense-System Maintenance Services	Defense Civil Preparedness Agency DOD	Funds for annual operating and maintenance costs of local C.D. communications systems; funds for training em personnel	Project Grants (Matching funds)	State and local C.D. organizations	Same as applicant	(Grants) FY '73: $1,425,732 FY '74: est. $1,642,000 FY '75: est. $1,700,000	FY '73: about 1,292 project applications submitted for approval	Communication systems maintenance Training C.D. personnel
12.321 Civil Defense-State and Local Supporting Systems Equipment	Defense Civil Preparedness Agency DOD	Purchase EMS equipment and communications for C.D. and other emergencies	Project Grants (Matching funds)	State and local C.D. organizations	Same as applicant	(Grants) FY '73: $2,214,698 FY '74: est. $4,000,000 FY '75: est. $4,000,000	FY '73: about 1,933 project applications approved	EMS equipment to establish an attack warning and communications system; Procure EMS equipment for rescue and training.
12.322 Civil Defense Contributions Project Loan Program	Defense Civil Preparedness Agency DOD	Provides for use of Federal excess personal property	Use of property, facilities, equipment	State and local C.D. organizations	Same as applicant	(Value of property loaned - original acquisition cost) FY '73: $35,000,000 FY '74: est. $30,000,000 FY '75: est. $30,000,000	FY '73: $30,000 worth of equipment loaned to all 50 states	

Table B-2. continued

Number/Title	Federal Agency	Objectives Uses	Type of Assistance	Applicant Eligibility	Beneficiary Eligibility	General Program Obligations	Program Accomplishments	EMS Subsystem
12.X01* Military Assistance to Traffic and Safety (MAST)	MAST, Health and Environment, Dept. of Defense	Provide air transport and related medical services to a community	Services	A community that 1) has a military base and 2) has communication hardware and a coordinated EMS system	Community victims	From Dept. of Defense training budget	Currently 22 sites participating	Transportation (air)
13.224 Health Services Development - Project Grants (Partnership for Health)	Health services Adm. PHS DHEW	Supports a full range of public health services in accordance with state comprehensive health planning	Project Grants (Share posts)	Any public or non-profit private agency; institution or organization	Same as applicant	(Grants) FY '73: $100,012,828 FY '74 est. $1,981,000 FY '75: est. $1,874,000	FY '74: 118 Neighborhood Health Centers in urban poverty areas	New health services programs must include EMS services and training as part of ambulatory care program
13.226 Health Services Research and Development - Grans and Contracts	HRA PHS DHEW	Research, development, demonstration and evaluation to improve health services	Project Grants Research Contracts (cost sharing)	States, poltcal subdivisions, universities, hospitals and other public or nonprofit private agency	Same as applicants	(Grants and Contracts) FY '73: $40,472,729 FY '74: est. $51,048,000 FY '75: est. $40,800,000	FY '74: Numerous research and demonstration projects being funded	Project designed to develop/evaluate ways of using manpower, equipment, facilities
13.228 Indian Health Services	HSA PHS DHEW	Provide inpatient and outpatient medical care to American Indians and Alaska natives	Provision of specialized services advisory services and counselling	Generally, Indians	Same as applicant	(Salaries and penses) FY '73: $176,850,356 FY '74: est. $202,052,101 FY '75: est. $227,758,000	FY '74: 107,000 Indian admission: 1,033,000 outpatient centers visits; 1,400,000 outpatient visits to hospitals	Full range of health services to Indian communities

*This number is not a Federal designation; it was composed for the *Program Guide* to enable inclusion of this activity.

127

Number/ Title	Federal Agency	Objectives Uses	Type of Assistance	Applicant Eligibility	Beneficiary Eligibility	General Program Obligations	Program Accomplishments	EMS Subsystem
13.235 Drug Abuse Community Service Programs	Alcohol, Drug Abuse, and Dental Health Adm. DHEW	Provides partial support of professional and technical personnel to staff community based aftercare services for drug dependent persons	Project grants Research contracts (cost sharing)	A community mental health center or affiliate; a public or non-profit private agency	Narcotic addicts and drug dependent persons	(Grants) FY '73: $83,663,218 FY '74: est. $108,227,000 FY '75: est. $82,859,000 (Contracts) FY '73: $24,612,188 FY '74: $25,747,000 FY '75: est. $12,900,000	FY '74: 27 Staffing grants: 228 drug abuse service projects	Staffing grants and drug abuse service projects
13.240 Mental Health - Community Mental Health Centers	Alcohol, Drug Abuse and Mental Health Adm. PHS DHEW	Financing of mental health services, including initial funds for professional and technical personnel	Project Grants	Construction grants available to state, political subdivision, public or non-profit private agency; staffing grants to areas providing five essential services	All persons who reside in the designated area	(Construction) FY '73: $8,306,144 FY '74: $34,250,000 FY '75: est. $0 (Staffing) FY '73: $165,000,000 FY '74: $155,513,000 FY '75: est. $172,053,000	FY '74: 210 construction grants 300 staffing grants planned	Manpower, other staffing grants for mental health centers

Table B-2. continued

Number/Title	Federal Agency	Objectives Uses	Types of Assistance	Applicant Eligibility	Beneficiary Eligibility	General Program Obligations	Program Accomplishments	EMS Subsystem
13.251 Alcohol Community Service Programs	Alcohol, Drug Abuse, and Mental Health Adm. PHS DHEW	To prevent and control alcoholism through comprehensive community services program; temporary staffing grants	Project Grants	Community Mental Health Center, public or nonprofit private organization affiliated with above, or located where no such center exists	Comprehensive services must be available to all alcoholic problem drinkers and their families who reside in the specified geographic area	(Grants) Staffing FY '73: $7,746,000 FY '74: est. $10,851,000 FY '75: est. $11,051,000	FY '74: expect to find 47 staffing agents; FY '75 expect about the same number	Other staffing grants; comprehensive services community mental health services
13.261 Family Health Centers	HSA PHS DHEW	To develop and provide health maintenance and treatment services on a prepaid capitation basis	Project Grants	Any public or non-profit private agency, institution, or organization	Population groups in areas of scarce health services	(Grants) FY '73: $10,178,087 FY '74: est. $13,000,000 FY '75: est. $13,000,000	FY '74: 39 projects awarded; 25 centers are operational, 14 being developed; FY '75: expect centers will serve 105,000 people	Manpower, Service Funds for development of treatment services, including training, ambulatory care benefits
13.284 Emergency Medical Services	Health Services Admin., Public Health Service, DHEW	Comprehensive EMS systems: feasibility studies, initial operations expansion, and improvement	Project Grants (some matching funds)	State, unit of general gov't., public entity, nonprofit private entities	Citizens of affected areas	FY '73: $0 FY '74: $17,000,000 FY '75: est. $17,000,000	FY '74: 135 for improvements	Practically all subsystems and components: personnel, training communic., transp., facilities, etc.

Table B-2. continued

Number/ Title	Federal Agency	Objectives Uses	Type of Assistance	Applicant Eligibility	Beneficiary Eligibility	General Program Obligations	Program Accomplishments	EMS Subsystem
13.285 Emergency Medical Services Systems Research	Health Resources Administration, Public Health Service DHEW	Direct costs and some indirect costs for research to provide useful information for technical assistance for EMS systems and to assist with policymaking at local, regional, and national levels	Project grants; Research contracts (must share costs, but no matching funds)	States, political subdivisions, universities, hospitals, and other public or nonprofit private organizations Grants also for individuals; contracts for profit organizations.	Same	FY '73: $0 FY '74: est. Section 304 - $8,000,000; Section 1205 - $3,333,000 FY '75: est. Section 1205 - $3,333,000	Not applicable - new program	Research in areas reaching practically all subsystems and components. (Areas covered include organizational analysis, new applications of medical devices, examination of sequence of pathopsychological changes following injury; studies of effectiveness of care; patient attitude and satisfaction studies; economic and financial studies; legal and policy related research; etc.)
13.305 Allied Health Professions- Special Project Grants	Health Resources Admin., Public Health Service, DHEW	Plan, establish, develop, demonstrate, or evaluate programs and techniques for training allied health personnel	Project Grants	Public or nonprofit organizations	Same	FY '73: est. $15,745,000 FY '74: est. $14,158,000 FY '75: est. not available	FY '74: 119 awards	Allied health professions (including EMIs)

130

Table B-2. continued

Number/ Title	Federal Agency	Objectives Uses	Type of Assistance	Applicant Eligibility	Beneficiary Eligibility	General Program Obligations	Program Accomplishments	EMS Subsystem
13.493 Vocational Education-Basic Grants to States	Office of Education, DHEW	Vocational education; construction, counselling, etc.	Formula grants-matching funds	State board for Vocational education	Individuals requiring vocational training	FY '73: $433,843,455 FY '74: $412,508,455 FY '75: preposed for inclusion in consolidated education grants legislative program	FY '74: $9,545,000 students served; est. 275 new and remodeled construction projects	Possibly all subsystems (e.g., EMT, dispatchers, allied health personnel, and other nonprofessional recognized and new and emerging occupations)
3.498 Vocational Education-Research	Office of Education, DHEW	Vocational education research, development, and personnel training programs, for youths; develop new careers (Youths-high school and follow up, e.g. community college)	Formula Grants Project grants (matching funds)	Formula grants: State boards for vocational education. Project grants: Institutions of higher education: public and private organizations, state boards	Broad field of vocational education	Formula grants: FY '73: $9,000,000 FY '74: $9,000,000 Project grants: FY '73: $9,000,000 FY '74: $9,000,000 All grants: FY '75: proposed for inclusion in consolidated education grants education program	FY '73: funds used for continued support and 425 career education projects. FY '74: Continuation of major emphasis in process	All subsystems (e.g., EMT, dispatchers, etc.)

131

Table B-2. continued

Number/Title	Federal Agency	Objectives Uses	Type of Assistance	Applicant Eligibility	Beneficiary Eligibility	General Program Obligations	Program Accomplishments	EMS Subsystem
13.714 Medical Assistance Program (Medicaid)	Social and Rehabilitation Service, DHEW	Provide financial assistance to states for medical assistance payments on behalf of recipients	Formula grants	State and local welfare agencies operating under an DHEW approved state plan and complying with other Federal regulations	Needy individuals eligibility determined by state in accordance with Federal regulations	(Grants) FY '73: $4,997,686,000 FY '74: est. $5,659,098,000 FY '75: est. $6,592,134,000	FY '74: est. 27,187,000 recipients FY '75: est. 28,566,000 recipients	ED visits Ambulance services
13.800 Medicare Hospital Insurance (Medicare)	Social Security Admin., DHEW	Hospital insurance to participating facilities for over 65 and specified others	Insurance	Over 65 (specifications)	Same	FY '73: $6,647,947,000 FY '74: est. $8,465,000,000 FY '75: est. $9,831,000,000	FY '75: 23,527,000 people protected	E.D.
13.801 Medicare- Supplementary Medical Insurance	Social Security Admin., DHEW	Insurance protection against health care costs, to physicians and other providers	Insurance	Over 65 (specifications)	Same	FY '73: $2,391,128,000 FY '74: $2,966,000,000 (est.) FY '75: est. $3,586,000,000	FY '75: est. 11,949,000 enrollees	E.D. transportation
14,128 Mortgage Insurance - Hospitals	Housing Production and mortgage credit/FHA, Dept. of Housing and Urban Development	Finance construction or rehabilitation of hospitals, includes major movalbe equipment	Guaranteed/ insured loans (max. mortgage: 90% of cost)	Licensed proprietary or private nonprofit institution	Persons needing services	FY '73: $100,443,000 FY '74: est. $156,260,000 FY '75: est. $123,020,000	FY '73: 15 project mortgages	E.D.

Table B-2. continued

Number/ Title	Federal Agency	Objectives Uses	Type of Assistance	Applicant Eligibility	Beneficiary Eligibility	General Program Obligations	Program Accomplishments	EMS Subsystem
14.701 Disaster Assistance	Federal Disaster Assistance Admin., Dept. of housing and Urban Development	To alleviate suffering and hardship from disasters	Project Grants; Use of property facilities, and equipment; provision of specialized services	State and local gov'ts. in declared disaster areas, owners of private non-profit medical care facilities, and individual disaster victims	Same	(Grants) FY '73: $486,188,000 FY '74: est. $533,588,000 FY '75: est. $100,000,000	FY '73: 53 disaster areas were declared involving 30 states	F.D. transportation Communication
14.702 State Disaster Plans and Programs	Federal Disaster Assistance Admin., Dept. of Housing and Urban Development	To improve disaster readiness and response capabilities. A state can apply for up to $250,000 a year for planning (no hardware) for disasters. After being declared a disaster area, FDAA will assist in obtaining help as needed (hardware, staff, etc.)	Project grants Formula and matching requirements	States	Same	FY '73: $351,000 FY '74: est. $518,000 FY '75: est. $1,478,000	FY '73: 25 states enrolled in program	A system as a whole

Table B-2. continued

Number/ Title	Federal Agency	Objectives Uses	Type of Assistance	Applicant Eligibility	Beneficiary Eligibility	General Program Obligations	Program Accomplishments	EMS Subsystems
16.502 Law Enforcement Assistance	Law Enforcement Assistance Admin., Dept. of Justice	To improve and strengthen all aspects of local law enforcement programs	Project grants; Formula grants	States with law enforcement planning agency and approved state plan	Operating law enforcement units of such states	FY '73: $536,750,000 FY '74: $536,750,000 FY '75: $536,750,000	FY '75: 20,000 subgrants active	Funds for shared county-wide/municipal communication system used for law enforcement and EMS
17.228 National On-the-job Training	Manpower Admin. Dept. of Labor	Occupational training for unemployed; can be used for reimbursement for instructors, admin. costs, supplies, supportive services, support for trainees, etc.	Project grants	National organizations with ability and desire to carry out program objectives	Unemployed or underemployed, age 16 or over, who cannot reasonably expect to secure full-time employment without training	FY '73: $15,600,000 FY '74: $14,000,000 FY '75: est. $14,000,000	FY '74: expected 22,000 training opportunities provided. Past contracts have included health service occupations.	Subsystems using allied health personnel (e.g., EMTs etc.), nurses, etc.
20.600 State and Community Highway Safety	National Highway Traffic Safety Administration, Federal Highway Admin., Dept. of Transportation	To provide coordinated national highway safety program, and reduce accidents, deaths, injuries, and damage; includes EMS (start up and some operations)	Formula grants	Approved state highway safety programs	Political subdivisions through state highway safety program	FY '73: $95,000,000 FY '74: $66,771,000 FY '75: est. $85,000,000	Reduction in traffic fatality rate, partially through improved EMS activities	Communic., transp.

Table B-2. continued

Number/Title	Federal Agency	Objectives Uses	Type of Assistance	Applicant Eligibility	Beneficiary Eligibility	General Program Obligations	Program Accomplishments	EMS Subsystem
21.X01* Revenue Sharing	Office of Revenue Sharing, Dept. of Treasury	Provision of revenue sharing funds for expenditures in priority areas, including health; capital and operating expenses	Revenue sharing funds	State; locality	State and local communities	FY '74: est. $6,700,000,000 FY '75: similar amount	FY '74: $477,100,000 Spent on "health" which consisted of 7% of general revenue expenditures	All (capital and operating)
23.004 Appalachian Health Demonstrations	Appalachian Regional Commission	Multicounty health demonstration projects for planning, facilities	Project Grants	States and through States health planning groups if project is designated as health planning; with publicly owned facilities or private nonprofit organizations	Recipients of health and child development services	(Grants) FY '73: $24,658,342 FY '74: est. $25,472,316 FY '75: est. $23,700,000	FY '73: 232 service projects in operation and 10 facilities under construction; FY '74: 265 service projects are estimated and an estimated 15 additional facilities will be under construction; FY '75: 187 service projects will be in operation and 10 additional facilities under construction	Communications, equipment, ambulances and training programs

*This number is not a Federal designation; it was composed for the *Program Guide* to enable inclusion of this activity.

Table B-2. continued

Number/Title	Federal Agency	Objectives Uses	Type of Assistance	Applicant Eligibility	Beneficiary Eligibility	General Program Obligations	Program Accomplishments	EMS Subsystem
59.X01* Small Business Loans	Small Business Administration	Loans available for a variety of situations for capital and operating expenses	Loans	For-profit, small business	Same	Varies for specific loan programs	Varies for specific loan programs	For-profit ambulance companies and hospitals
64.003 Education and Training of Health Service Personnel	Dept. of Medicine and Surgery, Veterans Administration	Provision of health services training in cooperation with academic institutions in medical and allied medical fields	Training (Direct payment for specified use)	Medical, dental, osteopathic, and nursing schools and other institutions of higher learning, medical centers, hospitals, and other public or non-profit bodies.	Trainee enrolled in qualifying institution	(salaries & expenses) FY '73: $138,130,000 FY '74: $154,159,000 FY '85: est. $180,861,000	FY '73: 65,528 persons received training FY '74: 67,000 persons expected to receive training	ED personnel; perhaps EMT training
64.011 Veterans Outpatient Care	Dept. of Medicine and Surgery, Veterans Administration	Outpatient medical and dental services to eligible vets	Provision of specified services	Specific requirements for eligible vets and their departments	Same	FY '74: $446,334,000 FY '75: est. $574,418,000	FY '73: total visits 10,858,491	Possibly F.D., ambulance service; contribution to local system coordination
64.018 Sharing Specialized Medical Resources	Dept. of Medicine and Surgery, Veterans Administration	To provide for exchange of or mutual use of specialized medical resources	Provision of specialized services	Medical schools, medical installations having hospital facilities, hospitals, or clinics	Patients of VA hospital or of eligible institution	(salaries & expenses) FY '73: $1,439,000 FY '74: $3,599,000 FY '75: est. $4,125,000	FY '73: 120 exchange of use and mutual use contracts were made	ED related. Perhaps transportation and/or communication

*This number is not a Federal designation; it was composed for the *Program Guide* to enable inclusion of this activity.

※ *Appendix C*

Selected References
and Resource Agencies

GUIDELINES FOR ORGANIZING AN EMS SYSTEM

1. *Developing Emergency Medical Services. Guidelines for Community Councils.* AMS, 1972. 15 pp. 20¢. American Medical Association, 535 North Dearborn St., Chicago, Ill.   60610.

2. *Economics of Highway Emergency Ambulance Services.* U.S. Department of Transportation. 63 pp. 65¢ . Superintendent of Documents, USGPO, Washington, D.C.   20402.

3. *Economics of Rural Ambulance Service in the Great Plains.* Agricultural Economics Report No. 308. 1975. 22 pp. U.S. Department of Agriculture, Economic Research Service, 500 12th St., S.W., Washington, D.C.   20250.

4. *Program Guidelines for Emergency Medical Service Systems.* HEW pub. No. (HSA) 75-2013 February 1975, 44pp, 85¢. Superintendent of Documents, USGPO, Washington, D.C.   20402, or from Regional DHEW Office.

5. *Safety Program Manual, Supplement I to Vol. II—Emergency Medical Services.* DOT, 1971. Department of Transportation, National Highway Traffic, Safety Administration, Washington, D.C.   20590.

6. *Planning and Implementing Community and County EMS Systems.* Southwest Research Institute, 1974. 84 pp. Available without cost. Texas Regional Medical Program, Inc., 4200 North Lamar, Suite 200, Austin, Texas 78756.

EMS COMMUNICATIONS

7. *911—The Emergency Telephone Number.* Franklin Institute Research Laboratories, 1973. 62 pp. $1.45. Stock No. 2205-0003. Superintendent of Documents, USGPO, Washington, D.C.   20402.

8. *Emergency Medical Services Communications Systems.* HEW, 1972. 38 pp. U.S. Department of Health, Education and Welfare, EMS Division, P.O. Box 911, Rockville, Md.   20852.

9. *A Guide for Hospital Participation in Emergency Medical Communications System.* A. H. A., 1973. 45 pp. $1.75. Catalog No. 1685. American Hospital Association, 840 North Lake Shore Drive, Chicago, Ill. 60611.

10. *Special Emergency Radio Service.* HEW, 1974. (Regulations creating an EMS category within SERS.) 19 pp. U.S. Department of Health, Education, and Welfare, EMS Division, P.O. Box 911, Rockville, Md. 20852.

11. *Federal Register,* July 16, 1974. Part III, "Federal Communications Commission, Medical Communications Services."

12. Federal Communications Commission. Public Notice No. 45715. *Emergency Medical Services (EMS) Systems Area Communication Plans.* Washington, D.C., Jan. 31, 1975.

13. *Federal Register,* Mr. 31, 1975. "Land Mobile Service."

14. *Communication Guidelines for Emergency Medical Services.* DOT, 1972. 74 pp. Superintendent of Documents, USGPO, Washington, D.C. 20402.

15. Office of Telecommunication Policy Bulletin No. 73-1, March 21, 1973. Office of Telecommunication Policy, Executive Office of the President, Washington, D.C. 20000.

TELEMETRY

16. *Telecommunications in Medicine (A Bibliography with Abstracts).* NTIS, 1975. 41 pp. Accession No. NTIS/PS-75/580/1GA. National Technical Information Service, U.S. Department of Commerce, 5285 Port Royal Road, Springfield, Va. 22161.

17. *A Report on a Biomedical Telemetry Standard for Emergency Medical Communications.* OTP, 1975. 54 pp. Office of Telecommunications Policy, Executive Office of the President, Washington, D.C. 20000.

18. *Telemetry Utilization for Emergency Medical Services System.* Georgia Institute of Technology, Health Systems Research Center, 1974. 76 pp. $4.75. National Technical Information Service, U.S. Department of Commerce, 5285 Port Royal Road, Springfield, Va. 22161.

19. Nagel, E. L., et al. "Telemetry of Physiologic Data," *Southern Medical Journal* (1968): 598-601.

20. *Federal Register,* June 10, 1975. "Notice of Inquiry and Rule Making, Docket No. 20488. Subject: Biomedical Telemetry Equipment; Standards for Design; Inquiry and Proposal.

21. Nagel, E. L., et al. *Telemetry and Physician/Rescue Personnel Communication,* U.S. Department of Transportation, NHTSA, Washington, D.C., Sept. 1971. 204 pp.

22. Communications/Telemetry Planning Guide, Wisconsin Emergency Medical Services Program, October, 1974; Division of Health, Wisconsin Division of Health and Social Services, Box 309, Madison, Wisconsin 53701.

23. Uhley, H. N. "Electrocardiographic Telemetry from Ambulances: A Practical Approach to Mobile Coronary Care Units," *American Heart Journal.* 80(1972):838-42.

24. Woodwark, G. M. *Monitoring of Ambulance Patients by Radio Telemetry,* *Canadian Medical Association Journal* 102(1970):1277-79.

25. Lambrew, C. T.; Schuchman, W. L.; and Cannon, T. H. "Emergency Medical Transport Systems: Use of ECG Telemetry," *Chest* 63(1973):477-82.

26. Lambrew, C. T. "The Experience in Telemetry of the Electrocardiogram to a Base Hospital," *Heart and Lung* 3(1974):756-64.

EMERGENCY CARDIAC CARE

27. *Proceedings of the National Conference on Standards for Cardiopulmonary Resuscitation (CPR) and Emergency Cardiac Care (ECC), 1973.* AHA, 1975. 264 pp. $3.20. American Heart Association, Distribution Section, 7320 Greenville Ave., Dallas, Texas   75231.

28. "Standards for Cardiopulmonary Resuscitation (CPR) and Emergency Cardiac (ECC)." (Supplement to *Journal of the American Medical Association,* Feb. 18, 1974.) 35 pp. American Heart Association, Distribution Section, 7320 Greenville Ave., Dallas, Texas   75231.

29. *Sudden Cardiac Death and the Onset of Myocardial Infarction.* Miami University, School of Medicine, Feb. 1974. 33 pp. $3.25. National Technical Information Service, U.S. Department of Commerce, 5285 Port Royal Road, Springfield, Va.   22161.

30. Graf, W. S., et al. "A Community Program for Emergency Cardiac Care." *Journal of the American Medical Association, JAMA,* Oct. 8, 1973, pp. 156-60.

31. Pantridge, J. F., and Geddes, J. S. "Mobile Intensive Care Unit in the Management of Myocardial Infarction. *Lancet* 2(1967):271.

32. Lewis, A. J., et al. "Pre-Hospital Cardiac Care in a Paramedical Mobile Intensive Care Unit," *California Med.* 117(1972):1-8.

33. *Pre-Hospital Emergency Cardiac Care.* (Subcommittee on Cardiac Emergencies, Committee on Emergency Medical Services, National Academy of Sciences.) *Para-Medical Journal* (Spring 1974). (*Para-Medical Journal,* Weamer Bldg. Rm. 23, Indiana, Pa.   15701.

34. Cobb, L. A., et al. "Pre-Hospital Coronary Care: The Tole of a Rapid Response Mobile Intensive Coronary Care System," *Circulation* 43(1971):139.

35. Grace, W. J. "The Mobile Coronary Care Unit and the Intermediate Coronary Care Unit in the Total Systems Approach to Coronary Care," *Chest* 58(1970):363-68.

36. Rose, L. B., and Press, E. "Cardiac Defibrillation by Ambulance Attendants," *Journal of the American Medical Association,* Jan. 3, 1972. pp. 63-68.

RURAL EMS

37. Lepper, R. L., et al. "An Overview of Rural EMS," *Emergency Medical Services* 4(1975):26-30.

38. *Health Services in Rural Areas: A Bibliography with Abstracts.* NTIS, 1974. 74 pp. National Technical Information Service, U.S. Department of Commerce, 5285 Port Royal Road, Springfield, Va.   22161.

39. *National Demonstration for Rural Emergency Medical Service: Final Report.* (Description of S.E. Ohio EMS project). NTIS, 1975. 300 pp. Document No. PB 246 398. National Technical Information Service, U.S. Department of Commerce, 5285 Port Royal Road, Springfield, Va.   22161.

40. *Rural Emergency Medical Services: Selected Bibliography.* DHEW, 1976. 24 pp. $1.10. Stock No. 017-026-00044-5. Superintendent of Documents, USGPO, Washington, D.C. 20402.

40a. Emergency Medical Services System Act of 1973; 93d Congress, Senate Report No. 93-397, Calender No. 373, September 18, 1973; Superintendent of Documents, Washington, D.C. 20402.

LEGAL ASPECTS OF EMS

41. *Evaluation of Legal Barriers to EMS Implementation.* Transactions Systems, Inc. Atlanta, Ga.: HEW 1974. 172 pp. Accession No. PB-244 326/5Ga. $6.25.

Appendix A. "Survey of Legislative Documents and Interviews with EMS Officials." Accession No. PB-243 725/9Ga. 622 pp. $15.25.

Appendixes B-F. "Survey of State, Territorial, Federal Legislation." 244 pp. Accession No. PB-244 318/2GA. $7.50.

National Technical Information Service, U.S. Department of Commerce, 5285 Port Royal Road, Springfield, Va. 22161.

42. *A Model Ordinance of Statutes Regulating Ambulance Service.* 15 pp. NSC, 1974. National Safety Council, 425 North Michigan Avenue, Chicago, Ill. 60611.

43. *State Statutes on Emergency Medical Services.* HEW, 1972. Stock No. 1725-0016. 192 pp. $1.50. Superintendent of Documents, USGPO, Washington, D.C. 20402.

EMS EVALUATION

44. *An Evaluation Methodology for Emergency Medical Services (EMS) Systems.* NATO, 1973. 198 pp. $3. National Technical Information Service, U.S. Department of Commerce, 5285 Port Royal Road, Springfield, Va. 22161.

45. *Methodologies for the Evaluation and Improvement of Emergency Medical Services Systems—Final Report.* Graduate School of Management, UCLA, July 1975. 569 pp. $13. Report No. DOT HS-801-648. National Technical Information Service, U.S. Department of Commerce, 5285 Port Royal Road, Springfield, Va. 22161.

46. *Model of the Risk of Death from Myocardial Infarction.* Shan Cretin, MIT Technical Report TR-09-74, MIT Technology Operations Research Center, 1974. 278 pp. Massachusetts Institute of Technology, Laboratory of Architecture and Planning, Room 4-209, Cambridge, Mass. 02139.

47. *Evaluation of EMS Systems Impact.* Transaction Systems, Inc. Atlanta, Ga., 1975. 25 pp. $3.25. Accession No. PB-243 714/3GA. National Technical Information Service, U.S. Department of Commerce, 5285 Port Royal Road, Springfield, Va. 22161.

48. Gibson, G. "Guidelines for Research and Evaluation of Emergency Medical Services," *Health Services Reports,* (March/April 1974):99.

49. *Development of a Minimum Data Set for EMS Patient Record Keeping.*

Macro Systems, Inc., Silver Spring, Md., 1974 (for HEW). Accession No. PB–243 822/4GA. 72 pp. $4.25.

Procedural Handbook: two volumes: Vol. I: Accession No. PB-243 781/2GA. $4.25. Vol. II: Accession No. PB-243 782/0GA. $5.25.

National Technical Information Service, U.S. Department of Commerce, 5285 Port Royal Road, Springfield, Va. 22161.

PUBLIC EDUCATION

50. *Consumer Education and Information Handbook for the EMS System.* AHSF, 1973. 29 pp. $2.50. Arkansas Health Systems Foundation, Southland Plaza Building, Suite 400, 6th & McKinley, Little Rock, Arkansas 72205.

51. *Attitudes and Perceptions of Groups Engaged in the Provision of Emergency Medical Services.* K. A. Stevenson and T. R. Willemain, 1974. 73 pp. Technical Report TR-11-74. Massachusetts Institute of Technology, Laboratory of Architecture and Planning, Room 4-209, Cambridge, Mass. 02139.

52. *Emergency Medical Services Consumer Education and Information.* Superior California Comprehensive Health Planning Association, 1974. 113 pp. Superior California CHP Association, 584 Rio Lindo Rd., Chico, California 95926.

53. *Emergency Medical Services—Consumer Education Manual.* California Regional Medical Program, 1975. $5.00. From: Publications Office, CRMP, 7700 Edgewater Drive #520, Oakland, Calif. 94261.

AGENCIES WITH ADDITIONAL INFORMATION

1. National Aeronautics and Space Administration
   OTDA, Code TN
   600 Independence Avenue, S.W.
   Washington, D.C. 20546
2. Department of Labor
   601 D. Street, N.W.
   Washington, D.C. 20213
3. Bureau of Medicine and Surgery
   Navy Department Code 72
   Washington, D.C. 20372
4. Federal Preparedness Agency
   General Services Administration
   Washington, D.C. 20405
5. Department of Health, Education and Welfare
   ADAHA, Room 18C-03
   5600 Fishers Lane
   Rockville, Maryland 20352
6. Division of Emergency Medical Services
   Room 320-6525
   Belcrest Road
   W. Hyattsville, Maryland 20782

7. Division of Health Services Administration
   22 South Green Street
   Baltimore, Maryland   21201
8. U.S. Department of Agriculture
   Room 242-E Administration Building
   14th and Independence Avenue, S.W.
   Washington, D.C.   20250
9. Veterans Administration
   Telecommunications Service
   Code 353
   810 Vermont Avenue, N.W.
   Washington, D.C.   20420
10. Law Enforcement Assistance Administration
    633 Indiana Avenue
    Washington, D.C.   20531
11. Veterans Administration
    (ECG) Ambulatory Care (113)
    810 Vermont Avenue, N.W.
    Washington, D.C.   20420
12. National Center for Health Services Resarch
    Health Resources Adminstration
    Room 15A-19
    5600 Fishers Lane
    Rockville, Maryland   20851
13 Federal Communications Commission
    2025 M Street, N.W.
    Washington, D.C.   20554
14. Division of Advanced Productivity Research and Technology
    National Science Foundation
    Washington, D.C.   20550
15. National Highway Traffic and Safety Administration
    NASSIF Building
    400 7th Street, S.W.
    Washington, D.C.   20590
16. FDA Bureau of Medical Devices (AFK 300)
    5600 Fishers Lane
    Rockville, Maryland   20852

Glossary

Access — The means of calling for emergency help.

Audio — Pertaining to audible frequencies (ca. 15–20,000 cycles per second).

ALI — Automatic location identification—a device for displaying the geographic location of an incoming telephone call.

ANI — Automatic number identification—a device for displaying the telephone number of an incoming call.

Base Station — A fixed transmitter and receiver.

Call Box — Roadside, push-button device for summoning help (usually police or fire).

CB — Citizens Band—a group of 40 VHF low-band frequencies for use by private citizens.

Central Dispatch — A point from which the ambulances of a region are dispatched.

CHANNEL — May be used to identify specific radio frequencies providing either a one-way or two-way communication.

Channel 9 — The CB frequency designated by the FCC as an emergency channel.

CMED — Central medical emergency dispatcher—a trained dispatcher at the EMS communications center.

Control console — Desk-mounted panel for controlling the operation of a radio station or communications center.

Crystal — Item that determines the exact frequency of a radio unit.

Decibel — Abbreviated dB. A unit of transmission gain or loss. A measure of relative power levels.

Dedicated line — A telephone line restricted to a particular (EMS) use.

Doctor call — A means of notifying a doctor of a medical emergency.

Doctor talk — Radio talk between a doctor and a rescue squad.

Duplex — A means whereby both communicating stations can simultaneously receive and transmit.

Duplexer — A device which, at the right time, automatically switches a single antenna from transmit to receive and vice versa.

ECG (or EKG) — Electrocardiograph. A visual display of electrical impulses generated by the heart.

ED — Emergency department, usually a receiving hospital.

800 number — An arrangement for toll-free calling to a specified number.

EMT — An emergency medical technician who has satisfactorily completed the 81-hour EMT course, or its equivalent.

Enterprise number — An advertised telephone number to be used toll free by the caller and requires the intervention of a telephone operator.

Evaluation — Assessment of a system's inventory, operational efficiency, and medical impact.

FCC — Federal Communications Commission, the agency responsible for allocating frequencies, licensing radio operators, and enforcing regulations.

Frequency — Hertz (cycles per unit of time)—radio frequencies are often measured in megahertz (millions of cycles per second), abbreviated MHz.

Geographic assignment — Allocation of frequencies by geographic area (as opposed to real-time allocation).

Good Samaritan laws — Laws protecting providers of emergency medical assistance from lawsuits resulting from such assistance.

Hotline — A landline always open for immediate communication for a specified purpose.

HMO — Health Maintenance Organization

Interface A point where a transition is made between modes of operation.

Interference — Undesired signals on a radio frequency from other radio transmitters or from other sources of electromagnetic radiation.

Intermodulation distortion — The combination of two signals to form a third, interfering signal.

Landline — Telephone line between geographically separate points.

MAST — Military Assistance to Safety in Traffic programs. Operate in some areas to provide military helicopters and medical corpsmen that may cooperate with civilian communities EMS system.

Med I to VIII — Eight pairs of UHF channels designated for EMS use.

Microwave link — A wide-band point-to-point transmission system. Microwave channels are able to carry a large number of simultaneous transmissions.

MICU — Mobile intensive care unit—a vehicle equipped for emergency cardiac care and other advanced life-saving techniques, and staffed by paramedics, emergency-care nurses, or physicians.

Mobile repeater — A fixed repeater station (as opposed to a vehicular repeater) for relaying transmissions from mobile transmitters.

Mobile unit — A vehicular radio unit.

Multiplex — A method of combining several messages for simultaneous transmission over a single channel.

Mutual aid agreement — An agreement between public-safety agencies to respond to requests for service beyond their jurisdictional boundaries.

911 — A toll-free telephone number for emergency calls to public safety centers.

Pager — Radio receiving device for alerting a physician, squad member, or other personnel, usually by a tone signal.

Paramedic — An EMT who has been trained in advanced live-saving techniques.

Phone Patch — A means of interfacing the telephone lines with a radio system.

Portable units — Radio units that can be carried by hand.

Provider — Person or organization responsible for providing emergency care.

PSAP — Public Safety Answering Point—a place to which all emergency calls are received, to be relayed to the appropriate emergency service.

QRU — Quick response unit—groups of local citizens, usually in remote areas, trained to provide first aid until an ambulance can arrive.

RCC — Resource communication center—the communications center for an EMS system.

Real-time allocation — Assignment of frequencies as they are needed at the time.

Relay — See Mobile and vehicular relay.

Repeater — See as Relay.

SERS — Special Emergency Radio Service—frequencies reserved for use in situations endangering life or property.

Simplex operation — Radio system allowing communication between two stations in only one direction at a time.

Skip interference — Abnormal signal projection causing interference.

Squelch — Receiver circuitry for suppressing unwanted radio signals or radio noise.

Telemedicine — Close-circuit TV between medical centers for patient care.

Terminal — A location within a communication system where data may be injected or removed. A point of connection in an electrical circuit.

Telemetry — Radio transmission of ECG and other vital signs.

Transceiver — Combination of transmitter and receiver equipment that uses some of the components jointly in both transmitting and receiving.

UHF — Ultra-high frequencies—frequencies in the 300–3000 MHz range.

Vehicular repeater — A repeater function incorporated in mobile equipment for relaying transmissions from portable transmitters.

VHF — Very high frequencies—those in the 30–300 MHz range.

WATS — Wide Area Telephone Service will provide, for a fixed monthly fee, a toll free service within a designated area.

Voting System — A system for processing receiver outputs to select the best received signal for use in the communication system.

Index

About the Authors

James E. McCorkle, Jr., P.E. has been developing public safety communications systems for state and local governments in the midwest for over 23 years. His development of consolidated communication centers for public access in reporting emergencies began in 1962. He has had extensive field experience in developing EMS communication systems at the local level. He has written many articles in the field of integrated electronic communication systems. He is a registered professional engineer, licensed in the State of Colorado, and a member of the National Society of Professional Engineers and the Professional Engineers of Colorado. Since 1972, he has been employed as a consulting engineer in private practice to state and local governments in the development of individual and integrated public safety communication systems.

Eugene L. Nagel, M.D. began his experience in the emergency medical service in the early 1960s, when he helped develop one of the first telemetry systems to be used clinically in the United States (City of Miami, Florida, fire rescue service, 1966-74). He is very active in bringing EMS to the people in the urban and rural areas through private and Federal assistance programs. He is a graduate of Cornell University in Electrical Engineering and worked for five years before entering medical training at Washington University, St. Louis, Missouri, and specialized training in anesthesiology at the Columbia Presbyterian School of Medicine. He has written many articles and monographs in the field of resuscitation and emergency medicine, and is currently Professor and Anesthesiologist-in-Chief at Johns Hopkins University, School of Medicine, Baltimore, Maryland.

Brig. Gen. Donald G. Penterman (Ret.) has been working with several National committees since 1960, assisting in bringing the communication system planning now evolving by direction of the Emergency Service Act of 1973. During 1968-72 he directed a research project on highway EMS that studied the 911 emergency telephone number system and utilizing CD radio for reporting highway surveillance. He was instrumental in the establishment of the MAST program. He is a graduate of the Industrial College of the Armed Forces, specializing in national security. He retired in 1973 as Brigadier General, having served in the U.S. Army and Army National Guard for a period of over 35 years. He is now serving as a Special Assistant to the Chancellor, University of Nebraska Medical Center.

Robert A. Mason was a member of the original team that developed the EMS concept for the Department of Health, Education and Welfare and the Department of Transportation. In 1962 he was responsible for developing one of the early EMS communication systems in Santa Clara, California. He is presently employed as a system engineer manager by Communication Enterprises Incorporated, Redding, California. He is a member of the Institute of Electrical and Electronic Engineers and National Association of Public Safety Communication Operators.